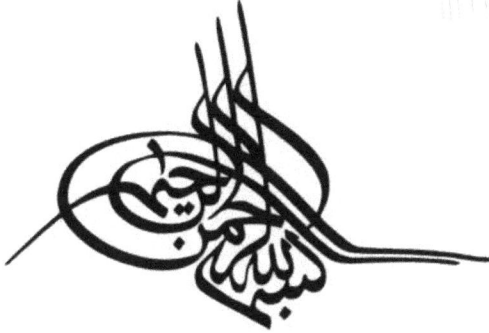

SILENCING
PAIN

MASTERING PAIN MANAGEMENT
FOR OPTIMAL PHYSICAL
REHABILITATION

Idris Hafiz, PhD

Disclaimer

This book is intended to provide general information on the topics covered. It is not meant to be used as a substitute for professional medical advice, diagnosis, or treatment. The reader should consult their healthcare provider with any questions regarding a medical condition or treatment. While the information contained herein is believed to be accurate and reliable, the publishing team and authors are not engaged in rendering medical, health, psychological, or any other kind of personal professional services through this book. Therefore, they cannot be held responsible for the accuracy or completeness of the information provided or for any errors, omissions, or results obtained from the use of such information.

The publisher and authors specifically disclaim any responsibility for any liability, loss, or risk, personal or otherwise, incurred as a consequence, directly or indirectly, of the use and application of any of the contents of this book. If medical or other expert assistance is required, the services of a competent professional should be sought to ensure that the reader receives appropriate and individualized care and consultation.

Idris Hafiz is a highly experienced clinical physiotherapist with a diverse and extensive background in both Canada and internationally. He holds a Bachelor of Physiotherapy from Gulf Medical University in the UAE, an MBA, and a (PhD) Doctorate in Physical Therapy from Atlantic International University in the USA. His advanced training includes fellowships in Orthopaedic Rehabilitation and Manual Therapy, and he is certified in Therapeutic Exercises.

Idris has further specialized in pain management, earning a Graduate Certificate from the University of Alberta, Canada, Faculty of Graduate Studies and Research (FGSR), Faculty of Rehabilitation Medicine. He also holds a Neuroplasticity Diploma and has completed the Pain Management Practitioner Program in the United Kingdom. Idris has participated in Explain Pain courses with the Neuro Orthopaedic Institute in Australia and has completed courses in the McKenzie Method of Mechanical Diagnosis and Therapy.

Throughout his career, Idris has worked in a variety of settings, including hospital-based physiotherapy, private clinics, sports medicine, and community-based rehabilitation services. This diverse experience has provided him with a comprehensive and nuanced perspective on physical therapy treatment, enabling him to address a wide range of patient needs effectively.

Dedicated to continuous learning, Idris integrates the latest evidence-based practices with a holistic approach to patient care. He is passionate about helping patients on their healing and recovery journeys, striving to ensure the highest standards in pain management and physical rehabilitation. His commitment to his patients and his field is evident in his ongoing pursuit of advanced training and his dedication to applying innovative and effective treatment strategies.

Idris's expertise and compassionate approach make him a highly respected and sought-after physiotherapist, committed to improving the quality of life for his patients through meticulous and personalized care.

Silencing Pain, Mastering Pain Management for Optimal Physical Rehabilitation

ISBN 978-1-0688731-2-6 (Hardcover)

ISBN 978-1-0688731-0-2 (eBook)

Designed by Waqar Nadeem

Edited by Pooja Yadav

www.silencingpain.com.

Pain, in its many guises, is an undeniable part of the human narrative. Whether transient or persistent, it leaves an indelible mark on our psyche, reminding us of our vulnerability yet simultaneously kindling our resilience. "Silencing Pain" is conceived from a pressing need to address this duality, particularly within the realm of physical rehabilitation.

Physical rehabilitation represents a path towards regaining what was lost—movement, function, or even a sense of self. However, this path is often strewn with the hurdles of pain, each demanding its own strategy and its own understanding. This book, then, serves as both a beacon and a manual, guiding its readers—whether they be patients, caregivers, or healthcare professionals—through the intricacies of pain and its management.

In "Silencing Pain," you will uncover the latest in pain management techniques and nuanced, holistic approaches that recognize physical rehabilitation as a journey of both the body and mind. Interspersed with real-life narratives, the chapters highlight the fortitude of those who've faced and overcome their pain, providing inspiration for others on a similar journey.

Beyond the clinical and therapeutic, this book delves into the emotional tapestry woven around pain. It offers solace, understanding, and strategies to manage pain and thrive in its presence. Drawing from years of research and firsthand experiences, the insights within these pages are both profound and pragmatic.

As you turn these pages, my hope is that "Silencing Pain" becomes more than just a guide—it becomes a companion—a testament to the human spirit, physical rehabilitation advancements, and the promise of a pain-free future.

With gratitude and optimism,

Idris Hafiz, *BPT, MBA, GC Pain, PhD*

Physical Therapist

Ottawa, Canada

From my early childhood memories, there has always been something strong and steadfast in my life, like a centuries-old tree with deep roots that nourishes the earth with wisdom, strength, and love. Although humble, this dedication is meant to honor those who have been faithful to my life.

The Pillars: My Parents

Each word I compose and each feeling I express reflects the lessons and values my guardians ingrain in me. They were mine, to begin with, instructors who instructed me not, as it were, to peruse words but too to get it their profundity. On days when doubt crept in, and the weight of ambition seemed unbearable, my mother's steadfast conviction held me back. They taught me to see setbacks as preparation for a comeback and failures as mere detours to success. My infinitely wise mother often spoke to me about resilience, determination, and the importance of staying true to yourself. She taught us the power of words to heal, inspire, and transform. My father had an immortal spirit and was the epitome of hard work. His example shows that success depends on processes, not goals. He taught me the essence of patience and the value of honesty.

The North Star: Fatima

More than just family, my oldest sister, Fatima, is a lighthouse in my life. Combining her grace with humility and strength, she has weathered the storms of her life with her quiet resilience. I have always admired her. She was my compass on this journey and guided me in the right direction. Fatima's constant support kept me upright whenever the world's weight bent my spine. Her stories of boldness, giggling within the confront of adversity, and immovable conviction within the control of her dreams formed my story.

This book, in this manner, isn't fair a result of my encounters and bits of knowledge, but moreover, the summit of the adore lessons and bequests that my family endowed me.

TABLE OF CONTENTS

THE HISTORICAL JOURNEY OF PAIN MANAGEMENT

"Healing is a matter of time, but it is sometimes also a matter of opportunity."
- Hippocrates

Synopses: *Dive into a captivating exploration of how societies across ages and continents have grappled with the universal experience of pain. From the ancient civilizations of Egypt and China, employing herbs and acupuncture, to the medieval theories of humour and the advent of modern anesthetics, this chapter offers a panoramic view of humanity's age-old quest to understand and alleviate pain. Uncover tales of pioneering thinkers and practices, some revolutionary and others best left in the past. Learn how evolving conceptions of the body, mind, and spirit have shaped pain management, laying the groundwork for today's multifaceted approaches. Through this journey, we'll recognize patterns of thought that have persisted and the innovations that have transformed the essence of pain treatment. Whether a testament to human resilience, a reflection of societal values, or the relentless pursuit of scientific knowledge, pain management's historical journey is a rich tapestry, revealing as much about our ancestors as about ourselves. Join me on this enlightening voyage as I chart the milestones, challenges, and breakthroughs that have defined the realm of pain management through the millennia.*

The history of pain management chronicles the evolution of medical practices, cultural beliefs, and methodologies devised to alleviate human suffering. This intricate narrative traverses various cultures, eras, and philosophical perspectives. As a consistent element of human existence since the outset of civilization, our understanding and approach to pain have witnessed considerable transformation. Here's a succinct overview:

Ancient and Pre-Modern Periods:

Ancient civilizations combined spiritual rites with naturalistic remedies for pain relief. Rituals and sacrifices were thought to placate deities, while early herbal treatments, notably opium, found favour among the Sumerians, Assyrians, and Egyptians. Hippocrates, the renowned Greek physician, championed a holistic medical perspective, emphasizing diet, exercise, and environment. Several societies documented the use of herbs like mandrake and henbane as pain relievers and alcohol for its numbing properties. Ancient China introduced methods such as acupuncture, a practice still prevalent today. Medical luminaries of the Islamic Golden Age, notably Ibn Sina (Avicenna), shed light on pain management, particularly emphasizing narcotics in his "The Canon of Medicine." The Renaissance period saw herbal solutions remain pivotal, but insights from the Islamic world and ancient cultures gradually reentered European medical discourse. In the 16th century, they heralded the advent of opium tinctures and laudanum, enhancing pain relief methodologies (Abdoli, Motamedi, & Zargaran, 2019).

18th and 19th Centuries:

The perception of pain started being viewed as a sensory experience. René Descartes, the French philosopher, introduced the idea of pain receptors and pathways. (Ho, 2007). The late 18th century saw nitrous oxide's discovery, propelling the advent of anesthesia, a boon for surgeries. Friedrich Sertürner, a German pharmacist, isolated morphine in the early 19th century, offering potent pain relief, albeit with emerging addiction issues. The mid-19th century marked the invention of the hypodermic needle, optimizing drug administration. (R, 1985)

20th century:

The late 19th-century creation of aspirin and the subsequent discovery of NSAIDs transformed pain management. The mid-20th century ushered in corticosteroids, effective in curbing inflammation and pain. Melzack and Wall's 1965 proposition of the gate control theory revolutionized pain perception understanding (Katz & Rosenbloom, 2015). The 1970s introduced patient-controlled analgesia (PCA) devices, allowing patients more autonomy in pain medication administration. (Macintyre, 2001)

Modern Era and Current Trends:

The late 20th century spotlighted aggressive pain management, marked by the rise of opioids for chronic pain. However, awareness of the addiction and overdose potential led to opioid use reassessment. Interdisciplinary pain management programs have gained prominence. Today, pain management emphasizes a holistic approach, combining physical, psychological, and emotional strategies. Techniques like spinal cord stimulation, deep brain stimulation, and biologic drugs like monoclonal antibodies are in vogue. There's a heightened focus on the synergy between the mind and body in pain management, elevating holistic treatments like mindfulness, yoga, and cognitive-behavioral therapy. Personalized treatment strategies, rooted in genetics and lifestyle, have become integral. (Meldrum, 2003)

Alternative treatments, from acupuncture to mind-body techniques, are gaining ground. Advancements like neurostimulation and implantable devices offer innovative pain management avenues. Today, pain management is a distinct medical specialty with an array of pain-relieving medications. Opioids, though effective, have raised addiction and overdose concerns. Interdisciplinary approaches and advances in neuroimaging have provided holistic, tailored pain relief solutions. (Rosenblum, Marsch, Joseph, & Portenoy, 2008)

Throughout history, pain perception and treatment shifts mirror advancements in medicine, societal attitude evolutions, and a growing emphasis on patient-focused care. The pursuit of efficient and empathetic pain management continues to mould medical practices, enriching the lives of those afflicted with pain. Despite progress, pain remains a multifaceted health challenge. Continuous research seeks to fine-tune pain management approaches, also delving into the societal and ethical dimensions of pain relief.

Pain phenomena encompass the intricate aspects of pain experience, from its root mechanisms and types to its causes and potential treatments. Delving into the neurobiology of pain means examining the channels and receptors in pain transmission, modulation processes, and the psychological facets of pain perception. Dr. Serge Marchand, a distinguished neurophysiologist, professor, and director at the Etienne-Le Bel Research Center of Sherbrooke University Hospital, has been instrumental in broadening our comprehension of these elements. In "Phenomena of Pain," Dr. Marchand provides a comprehensive insight into pain, unravelling its complexities through a systematic structure that covers its many facets, mechanisms, and therapeutic approaches (Marchand, 2014). While many types of pain can be eradicated entirely, others might only be managed. The approach often depends on the individual, the cause of their pain, and the available treatments. Regardless, the goal is always to improve the individual's quality of life, whether eradicating or managing the pain effectively. Today, the persistence of poor pain control, especially for patients with chronic pain, despite the availability of powerful analgesics and supplementary treatments, is perplexing. Bourke examines possible causes from both sufferers' and clinicians' perspectives and concludes,' *it does not emerge naturally from physiological processes, but in negotiation with social worlds*' (Seamark, 2015).

Key Message:

Understanding the historical journey of pain management empowers patients with chronic pain by providing valuable insights into the evolution of treatments, enhancing informed decision-making, fostering hope, improving communication with healthcare providers, validating their experiences, and supporting advocacy efforts. This knowledge enriches patients' perspectives and engagement in their care, leading to better chronic pain management.

Reflection Exercise:

True or False:

1. Opioids are no longer used in modern pain management due to their addiction potential.

2. The gate control theory suggests that pain perception is purely a psychological experience.

3. Personalized treatment strategies in pain management are rooted in genetics and lifestyle.

4. For Patients: How do you perceive and understand your pain, and in what ways can exploring the underlying mechanisms and psychological aspects of your pain experience help you better manage it?

Response: _____

_____

_____

5. For Health Providers: How can a deeper understanding of the neurobiology and psychological facets of pain enhance your approach to treating patients, and what strategies can you employ to address both the physiological and social factors influencing pain perception and management?

Response: _____

_____

_____

Answers:

1. False

2. False

3. True

THEORIES OF PAIN

"There are no incurable diseases — only the lack of will. There are no worthless herbs — only the lack of knowledge."

Avicenna (Ibn Sina)

Synopses: *In this chapter, we delve into the intricate realm of pain perception, unravelling the foundational theories shaping our comprehension of this universally encountered phenomenon. We explore the philosophical dilemmas and scientific discoveries that have sought to unravel pain's essence, origins, and effects on the human mind. We navigate through groundbreaking theories on pain perception, from the transformative Gate Control Theory, revolutionizing our understanding of nerve impulses, to the Biopsychosocial Model, underscoring the interconnectedness of the body, mind, and society. Discover how these notions not only enlighten our understanding of pain engineering but also influence contemporary pain management and therapy strategies. As we scrutinize theories conceptualizing pain as a multifaceted interweaving of psychological, social, and environmental elements, not merely a physical experience, we invite readers to reevaluate their preconceived notions. "Theories of Pain" aims to offer readers extensive insight into discussing pain, blending science, philosophy, and therapeutic practice into a cohesive narrative about one of the most studied yet least understood human experiences. Brace yourself for an intellectually stimulating journey through one of the most intricate aspects of human existence, challenging and expanding your understanding of pain.*

Throughout human history, the perception of pain, with its uncanny ability to protect and torment, has been subject to intense scrutiny and contemplation. Its enigmatic nature has provoked theories ranging from the mystical to the empirical, each attempting to demystify this universal experience. In this chapter, "Theories of Pain," we journey through time and thought, exploring the myriad frameworks that have sought to define and understand pain.

From the ancient civilizations that viewed pain through a spiritual lens, seeing it as a divine message or a malevolent curse, to the Renaissance thinkers who began to connect pain with the physical body, and onto the modern era, where neuroscientists delve into the intricate web of neurons and synapses, our understanding has been in constant flux. Each era, each culture, and each pioneering thinker has added a layer to our comprehension and, sometimes, paradoxically, to our confusion.

"Theories of Pain" is not purely an academic exploration but a narrative highlighting the interplay between science, philosophy, culture, and individual experience. As we dive into various theories, we will confront challenging questions: Is pain purely a biological response? How do psychology and society influence our perception of pain? And as we delve into the future, how might technology and new discoveries reshape our understanding?

Join us in this intellectual adventure as we navigate the intricate labyrinth of theories that have attempted to capture the essence of pain, enriching our collective understanding of this most human of experiences. Through this exploration, we aim to inform and provoke reflection, inspire curiosity, and foster a deeper appreciation for the multifaceted nature of pain.

Pain is a complex and multifaceted experience that is both sensory and emotional. Over time, various theories have been proposed to explain the mechanisms underlying pain perception. Here are some of the prominent ones:

1. Specificity Theory:

Max Von Frey formulated the specificity theory of pain in 1895. This is one of the oldest theories of pain. It postulates that specific pain receptors in the body send signals to a pain center in the brain when stimulated. It assumes a direct relationship between the intensity of the stimulus and the intensity of the pain. This theory asserts a distinct region in the brain devoted solely to pain perception, similar to areas for vision and hearing. According to Von Frey, unique nerve endings in the skin relay pain signals. These signals are then directed through specialized channels to a designated "pain center" in the brain, resulting in the experience of pain.

However, the validity of the specificity theory has been challenged over time. A prime example is phantom limb pain, where individuals who've lost a limb still feel pain originating from the absent limb. This phenomenon contradicts the specificity theory, as no physical source sends signals in such cases (Moayedi, Davis, & Davis, 2013).

Furthermore, the phenomenon of using hypnosis as anesthesia presents another challenge to this theory. Remarkably, surgeries can take place under hypnosis, causing considerable tissue damage, yet patients don't report any pain, questioning the accuracy of Von Frey's perspective (Hammond, 2008). Although hypnosis can block the perception of pain, the body might still have a physiological response to injury or trauma. For instance, a patient might not feel pain during a procedure but still experience inflammation or other responses afterward.

2. Pattern Theory:

This theory, sometimes known as the Intensity Theory, emerged as an alternative to the Specificity Theory of pain. While the Specificity Theory posits that specific pain receptors and pathways are dedicated exclusively to transmitting pain signals, the Pattern Theory proposes a different mechanism for pain perception. It suggests that pain is not caused by specific pain receptors but rather by the frequency or pattern of signals sent to the brain. In this theory, any nerve can transmit a pain signal if stimulated intensely enough (Moayedi, Davis, & Davis, 2013).

Although the Pattern Theory offers an alternative view to pain perception, it also has limitations. For instance, it doesn't entirely explain why different types of stimuli (e.g., thermal, mechanical, or chemical) can produce distinct pain qualities. Nor does it account for more complex pain phenomena, like phantom limb pain or the modulatory effects of psychological processes on pain perception.

The Pattern Theory and Specificity Theory represent earlier attempts to understand the complex nature of pain. While both offer valuable insights, modern pain science has evolved to encompass more integrative models, like the Gate Control Theory and Biopsychosocial Model, which combine elements from both theories and integrate additional physiological and psychological components (Moayedi, Davis, & Davis, 2013).

3. Gate Control Theory:

This theory, proposed by Melzack and Wall in the 1960s, suggests that the spinal cord contains a "gate" mechanism that prevents pain signals from reaching the brain. This theory integrates both physiological and psychological components of pain, suggesting that cognitive and emotional processes can modulate pain perception (Moayedi, Davis, & Davis, 2013). This theory revolutionized our understanding of pain by highlighting the interaction between the nervous system and the brain in pain perception. This theory presents a more complex view of pain than previous models, such as the Specificity or Pattern theories.

The clinical implications of this theory are evident in TENS (transcutaneous electrical nerve stimulation) therapy, which offers relief for certain pain patients based on this approach (DeSantana, Walsh, Vance, Rakel, & Sluka, 2008). The TENS device employs electrical pulses to stimulate specific nerve fibres, thereby alleviating pain. This principle is also observed in distraction techniques, where pain perception can be reduced due to the brain's regulatory influence. Additionally, emotional states play a role in pain intensity, with positive emotions lessening pain and negative emotions intensifying it. Although the Gate Control Theory has provided valuable insights and influenced pain management strategies, it is just one piece of the puzzle of understanding pain. More recent perspectives consider a broader range of factors, including cognitive, emotional, and social dimensions (Mendell, 2014).

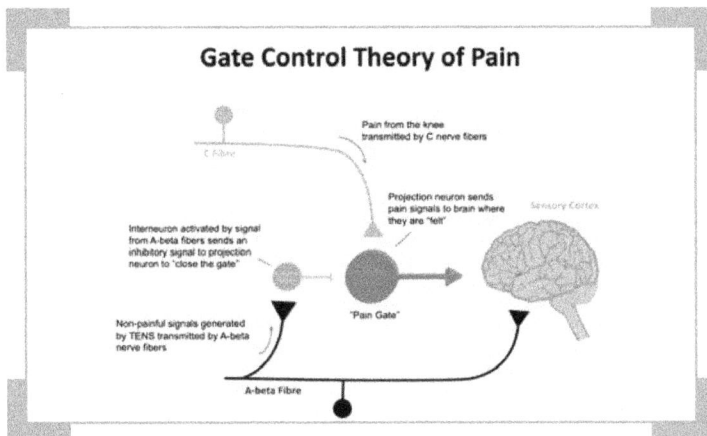

Gate Control Theory of Pain

4. Neuromatrix Theory of Pain:

This theory, proposed by Ronald Melzack in the 1990s, posits that pain is not merely a result of direct sensory input but is an output constructed by the brain. This theory developed as an extension of the Gate Control Theory. Central to the theory is the "neuromatrix," a network of neurons in the brain that processes various inputs, including emotional and cognitive factors, to produce the pain experience. This theory accounts for phenomena like phantom limb pain and emphasizes the brain's role in modulating pain perception. It suggests that pain management requires a multidisciplinary approach and offers insights into understanding and treating chronic pain. The theory highlights the brain's adaptability, suggesting interventions can reshape pain patterns (Melzack, 2005).

5. Biopsychosocial Model of Pain: This approach to understanding pain views it as a dynamic interplay between biological, psychological, and social. This model suggests that pain is not just a physical sensation but is also influenced by emotions, beliefs, social environment, and experience factors (Megan Pomarensky, Luciana Macedo, & Lisa C. Carlesso, 2022). Unlike traditional models that focus primarily on physiological processes, the biopsychosocial model emphasizes the complex interplay between the mind, body, and social environment in the experience of pain. Considering the intricate nature of chronic pain, adopting the biopsychosocial approach would be advantageous (Dwyer, et al., 2016).

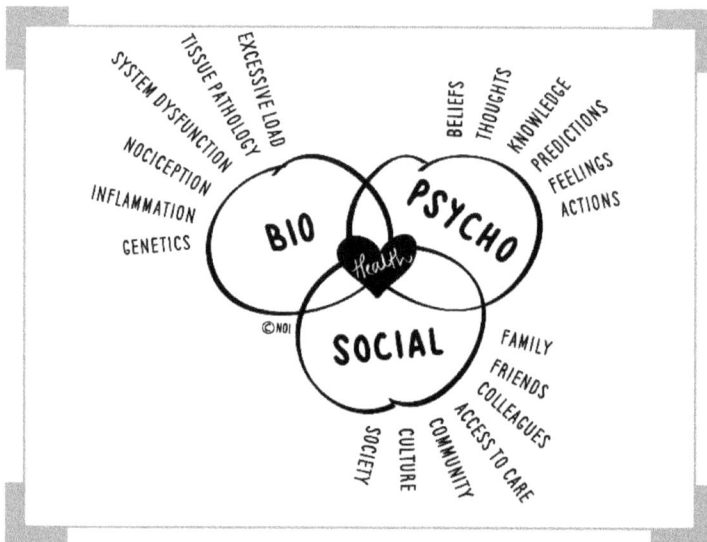

6. Central Sensitization: This theory proposes that persistent pain can result from the central nervous system becoming overly responsive or sensitized to pain signals. This can lead to conditions like fibromyalgia, where pain is felt even in the absence of a clear external cause (Cagnie, et al., 2014).

7. Descending Modulatory System (DMS): This theory posits that the brain has an internal system that can upregulate or downregulate pain signals. This system can either amplify or dampen pain based on various factors such as emotions, attention, and expectations. Key brain regions involved include the periaqueductal gray, the rostral ventromedial medulla, and the dorsal reticular nucleus. Dysfunctions in the DMS can contribute to chronic pain, as constant amplification or compromised inhibition leads to prolonged pain. Its understanding aids in the development of pain management strategies, both medicinal and non-pharmacological, by targeting its mechanisms (Bannister, 2019)

8. Fear-Avoidance Model: This is more of a behavioural theory. It suggests that individuals who interpret pain as a threat may become fearful and avoid activities that they associate with pain. This avoidance can lead to disability and chronic pain (Wong, et al., 2015). The Fear-Avoidance Model offers a comprehensive framework for understanding the transition from acute to chronic pain, emphasizing the interplay between cognitive processes, emotional responses, and behavioural outcomes. The model also highlights the value of early intervention. By addressing catastrophizing thoughts and fears early on, healthcare professionals can potentially prevent the development of chronic pain syndromes (Wilson JM, 2023) .

It's important to note that no single theory can capture the entirety of pain's complexity. Instead, these theories offer lenses through which we can understand different pain perception and management aspects. Our understanding of pain will likely evolve as research continues, leading to more comprehensive and integrative models.

Key Message:

Understanding the theories of pain equips patients with chronic pain with crucial insights that enhance their comprehension of pain, empower them with knowledge, and improve communication with healthcare providers. This knowledge supports personalized treatment plans, fosters effective coping strategies, reduces stigma, provides hope, aids in self-advocacy, promotes a holistic approach to care, and validates their experiences, leading to more effective pain management and overall well-being.

Reflection Exercise:

Use the following questions as a guide for your reflection. Write your responses in the space provided or in a separate document.

1. Reflect on your own understanding of pain. How have the theories discussed in this chapter changed or enhanced your perspective on pain management?

Response: _____

_____

_____

2. Consider a situation where you experienced pain. How might the theories of pain help explain your experience and guide you toward effective management strategies?

Response: _____

_____

_____

3. How can understanding the multifaceted nature of pain improve communication between patients and healthcare providers? Reflect on the importance of this understanding in creating personalized treatment plans.

Response: _____

_____

_____

4. How has the Gate Control Theory changed your perspective on the nervous system and brain interaction in pain perception?

Response: _____

_____

_____

5. Reflect on the practical applications of this theory, such as TENS therapy and distraction techniques. How do you view these methods now?

Response: _____

_____

_____

6. *For Patients: How do your thoughts and feelings about pain influence your daily activities, and what steps can you take to address any fears that might lead you to avoid certain activities?*

Response: _____

_____

_____

7. *For Health Providers: How can you help patients recognize and address their fears related to pain, and what strategies can you implement to prevent these fears from contributing to chronic pain development?*

Response: _____

_____

_____

Idea:

Reflecting on the theories of pain provides a deeper appreciation of the complexity of pain perception and management. Use your insights from this exercise to inform your future interactions with healthcare providers and to explore more effective pain management strategies.

DECIPHERING PAIN

*"Your pain is the breaking of the shell that
encloses your understanding."*

Kahlil Gibran

Synopses: In the enchanting weave of words titled "Deciphering Pain," we beckon you into the labyrinthine world of pain — a realm universal in its reach yet deeply intimate in its touch. Embark on a soulful journey to the core of human experience, where we unravel pain's multi-faceted tapestry. From the electric hum of neurons to the heart's silent screams, we delve into the brain's sophisticated ballet with distress signals, underlining the profound interplay of senses and intellect. We don't stop there; we tread further into the often-misty realms of the psyche and societal constructs, acknowledging that our pain narratives are etched just as much by cultural scripts as individual soul stories. Yet, how does one capture the enormity of pain? How do we chart its elusive shades? From rudimentary charts to the vanguard of brain scans, our attempt to pin down pain's essence is a saga in itself. But let's be clear, "Deciphering Pain" isn't just a scholarly odyssey; it's an ode — an ode to every tear shed, every grimace held back, and every heart that's ever ached. This chapter seeks to resonate with your soul through evocative tales and stirring musings, offering a panoramic view of pain. So, take your hand, dear reader. Dive deep, wander wide, and traverse this profound mosaic of life, feeling, and mystery together.

Pain — it's an age-old dance, a tango between the heart and flesh. This relentless partner has held humanity in a tight embrace from our very first steps, serenading us with both bitter and invaluable lessons. Sometimes, it's a gentle caress, a nudge towards caution; other times, it's a tempestuous storm, leaving scars and tales in its wake. In

"Deciphering Pain," we're setting sail into this tempest, searching for the lighthouse amidst its chaos.

We'll traverse time itself, from the whispered remedies of ancient shamans to the sterile yet hopeful halls of modern-day labs. While our grasp on pain has metamorphosed, darting between enlightenment and oblivion, our relentless pursuit to decode its enigma has never waned. What sparks this fire within? Why does this intricate dance echo so deeply within our psyche? And can we ever lead in this ever-present dance?

But, my dear reader, this chapter isn't just a foray into the annals of science. Oh no, it's a soulful ballad. As we dissect the sinews of pain's biology, venture into its psychological mazes, and meander through its cultural imprints, we'll also grapple with the heavier questions – the kind that lingers long after the last page is turned. What does pain reveal about our essence, boundaries, and boundless horizons?

So, pull up a chair, pour a cup of contemplation, and let's wade through this intricate tapestry together. "Deciphering Pain" isn't just about understanding; it's about reverence. Through these words, we strive to illuminate the dim corners, offering insights, solace, and a touch of awe for one of existence's most profound enigmas.

1-NAVIGATING THE MULTILAYERED LANDSCAPE OF DISCOMFORT:

This section delves into the varied dimensions of pain, acknowledging that pain isn't just a singular experience but a multi-faceted phenomenon that intertwines with our physical, emotional, and psychological states.

Let's start by understanding that "physical pain" and "pain mechanisms" are not the same thing, but they are closely related concepts. Let's differentiate the two:

Physical pain refers to the actual sensation of discomfort or distress that an individual perceives, often due to injury, disease, or some form of bodily harm. It can manifest in various ways, such as sharp, dull, throbbing, aching, burning, or stinging sensations, among others. Examples: A cut on your hand, a broken bone, or a headache would be instances of physical pain.

Pain mechanisms refer to the underlying biological and physiological processes that produce and modulate pain sensation. These mechanisms involve complex interactions between peripheral tissues, nerves, the spinal cord, and the brain.

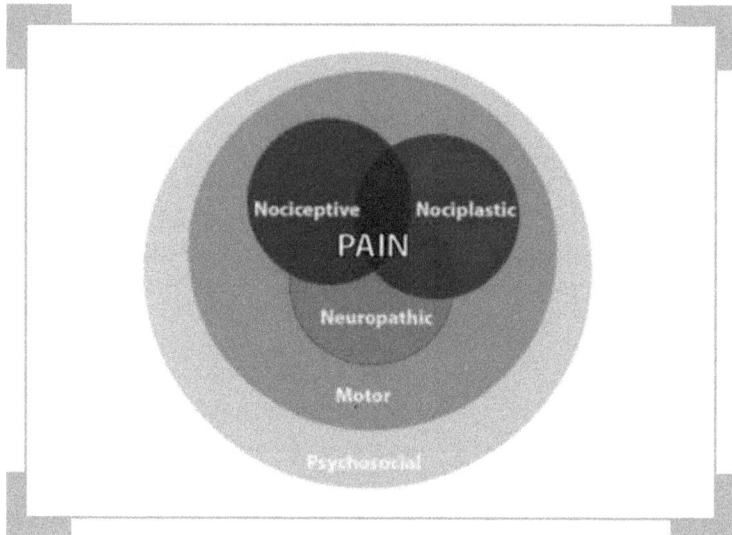

The International Association for the Study of Pain (IASP) is a global pain science and education leader. Their definitions and classifications play a crucial role in shaping how pain is understood and treated worldwide. IASP had recently revised its definition of pain. According to the IASP, pain is: "An unpleasant sensory and emotional experience associated with or resembling that associated with actual or potential tissue damage." This definition emphasizes not only the sensory aspect of pain but also the emotional dimension, highlighting the subjective nature of pain.

Regarding pain mechanisms, the IASP classifies pain into three main categories based on its origin:

Nociceptive Mechanism: Guardians of the Body:

Nociception, derived from the Latin "nocere," meaning "to harm," refers to the body's sensory response to potentially harmful stimuli. The body's early warning system is designed to detect and react to threats. The primary agents in this defence system are the nociceptors. This chapter delves into the intricacies of the nociceptive mechanism and how it safeguards the body.

Nociceptors: The First Responders

Nociceptors are specialized sensory receptors found throughout the body, particularly in the skin, muscles, joints, and some internal organs. Unlike other sensory receptors that respond to light touch or temperature, nociceptors are activated by stimuli that have the potential to cause damage.

Thermal Nociceptors: Activated by extreme temperatures. For example, when you touch a hot stove, the thermal nociceptors send signals of potential harm.

Mechanical Nociceptors: Respond to intense pressure or mechanical deformation, like pinching or crushing injuries.

Chemical Nociceptors: Sensitive to chemical substances released during tissue damage or inflammation, such as bradykinin, prostaglandins, and histamine.

Polymodal Nociceptors: These are versatile and respond to multiple types of noxious stimuli, whether thermal, mechanical, or chemical.

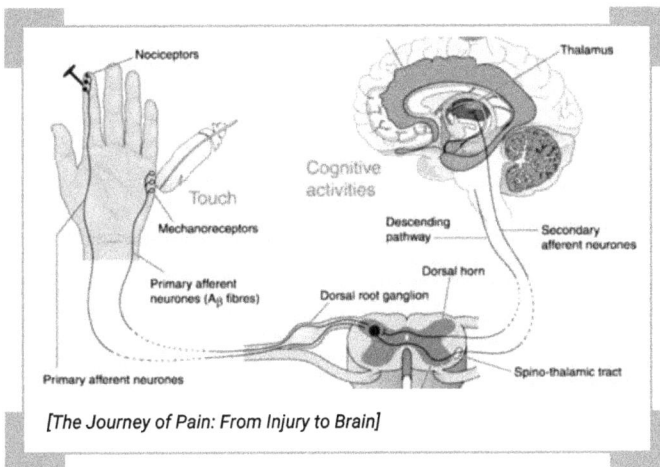

[The Journey of Pain: From Injury to Brain]

The Journey of Pain: From Injury to Brain

Upon activation, nociceptors transmit signals along nerve fibres, specifically Aδ and C fibres, towards the central nervous system. These fibres differ in their conduction speeds and the type of pain they relay:

Aδ fibres are thin, myelinated fibres that rapidly transmit sharp, acute pain.

C fibres: Unmyelinated and transmit dull, aching pain more slowly.

The pain signals travel up the spinal cord, passing through various neural gates and pathways, ultimately reaching the thalamus in the brain. From there, they are relayed to multiple brain regions responsible for interpreting the sensory and emotional aspects of pain.

Reflex Arcs: The Body's Quick Defense

Even before the brain consciously registers pain, the body often reacts. This rapid response is thanks to reflex arcs, neural pathways that bypass the brain for swift action. For instance, when touching something hot, the swift retraction of the hand results from a reflex arc in action.

Nociception and Inflammation: A Protective Duo

When tissue is damaged, a cascade of inflammatory responses is activated. This inflammation can further stimulate nociceptors, amplifying pain signals. This heightened sensitivity, known as hyperalgesia, ensures that the individual protects the injured area, allowing it time to heal.

The nociceptive mechanism, while often associated with pain discomfort, is fundamentally a protective system. It ensures that threats are promptly detected, interpreted, and responded to. By understanding this intricate network of receptors, fibres, and neural pathways, we appreciate the body's innate ability to shield itself from harm.

Neuropathic Mechanism: A Tale of Crossed Wires

In the vast, intricate tapestry of the human body, threads of nerves weave stories of sensations, from the gentlest of touches to the sharpest of pains. But what happens when these threads fray or tangle? Enter the realm of neuropathic pain, where the very messengers of sensation betray us, turning whispers into screams and shadows into spectres.

Amidst the bustling city of Neuronville, the nerve fibres acted as diligent messengers, transmitting tales of the world outside to the brain's grand hall. But some stories began to change, not from the world outside, but from the messengers themselves. These were tales not of external threats but of internal betrayals.

The Origins of the Distorted Tales

The paths of Neuronville weren't always safe. Accidents on the highways, like traumatic injuries, sometimes severed the threads. Diseases like diabetes, acting like saboteurs, eroded the fibres over time. Then, there were invaders like the shingles virus, which left destruction in its wake. And sometimes, even removing a part of the city, akin to amputation, led to ghostly tales of limbs that were no longer there.

Symptoms: The Echoes of Distress

The tales these compromised nerves told were unlike any other. They spoke of searing fires and biting cold, electric jolts shooting through the streets and a heightened sensitivity where even the gentlest breeze felt like a storm. The once-trusted messengers were now suspected of treachery.

The Underlying Chaos

As investigators delved deeper, they discovered the chaos within. Some nerve endings had become hyper-sensitive, magnifying every sensation. The central stations, where messages were processed, began amplifying tales out of proportion. Some nerve fibres, damaged in previous incidents, began sending false alarms and stories with no basis. And amidst all this, the glial cells, once the silent supporters, added to the mayhem by fueling the fires of inflammation.

As the sun sets on Neuronville, one can't help but marvel at the delicate balance that sustains this city. The tale of neuropathic pain is not just of crossed wires but of resilience, of seeking solutions amidst chaos, and of the eternal hope that even in a world gone awry, balance can be restored.

Nociplastic Mechanism: The Enigma of Altered Perception

4. Nociplastic pain: This is a relatively newer term in the pain classification realm and is significant in understanding pain mechanisms (IASP, n.d.). In the vast world of pain, where every twinge and ache tells a story, a relatively new protagonist has emerged on the scene: nociplastic pain. Unlike its well-known counterparts, nociceptive and neuropathic pain, which arise from clear tissue damage or nerve injury, nociplastic pain is more enigmatic.

Imagine the body's pain signalling system as a grand orchestra. In most scenarios, every instrument plays in harmony, reflecting the damage or disturbance in the body. But in the case of nociplastic pain, the orchestra begins to play an intensified or distorted tune, even when there is no clear reason to do so. It's as if the conductor — the central nervous system — has become overly sensitive, amplifying every note.

This mysterious kind of pain doesn't always correlate with visible injuries. People with conditions like fibromyalgia or irritable bowel syndrome, for instance, often bear the brunt of this erratic orchestra. Their pain isn't necessarily a direct result of observable tissue damage;

it's the result of a system in disarray processing pain signals differently—results from a retrospective "real world" data analysis of fibromyalgia patients.

Pain is not the major determinant of quality of life in fibromyalgia (Offenbaecher, 2021).

Understanding nociplastic pain is like unravelling a complex musical score. It requires keen attention to nuances and, most importantly, an acceptance that not all pain is as straightforward as a simple cause and effect. Addressing it means fine-tuning the body's orchestra, restoring harmony and balance to those who suffer.

Recognizing nociplastic pain is crucial for the appropriate management and treatment of pain, especially in cases where traditional interventions targeting tissue damage or inflammation might not be effective. Treatment often requires a multi-faceted approach, combining physical therapy, pain education, cognitive-behavioural therapy, and sometimes pharmacological interventions tailored toward modulating pain perception.

In summary, while "nociceptive" and "neuropathic" pain has been the primary classifications for many years, the introduction of "nociplastic pain" addresses a subset of pain conditions where the primary issue is altered nociception itself, rather than a direct response to tissue damage or nerve injury. It highlights the intricate nature of pain and the necessity for nuanced understanding and treatment strategies.

2. FROM SENSATION TO PERCEPTION: UNRAVELING THE MYSTERIES OF PAIN:

In a study conducted by The International Journal of Psychophysiology in 2019 involving Gulf War Veterans, researchers investigated how anticipating pain affects the brain, especially among those with chronic musculoskeletal pain (CMP). They exposed 61 Veterans (30 with CMP and 31 healthy) to non-painful thermal stimuli while monitoring brain reactions using fMRI. Participants also rated the perceived pain. The findings revealed that certain brain areas, like the cingulate cortex, showed altered activity when anticipating pain. Moreover, Veterans with CMP responded differently in the middle temporal gyrus compared to healthy Veterans. This study highlights the significance of pain anticipation in understanding brain responses, particularly in CMP patients (Jacob B. Lindheimer, 2019).

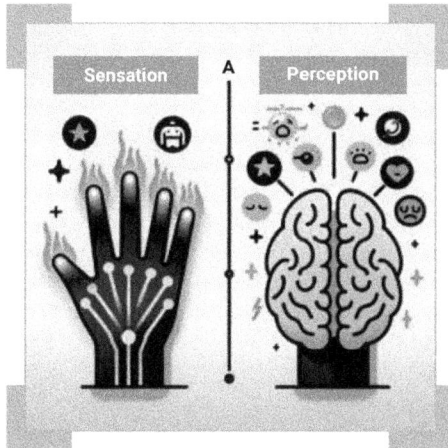

Let's delve deeper into the transition from sensation to pain perception, dissecting the stages, processes, and complex interplay of factors that turn a simple sensory input into the rich experience we recognize as pain. This will provide a more comprehensive and relatable understanding of the transition from sensation to pain perception.

1. Sensation: The Primary Alert

- Nociceptors: Imagine walking barefoot on a beach. The sand is warm, but as you step on a sharp shell, specific sensors in your foot (nociceptors) sound the alarm.

- Activation Thresholds: If the sand had been just mildly warm or the shell's edge smooth, your nociceptors would remain quiet. But crossing a certain threshold – the sharpness of the shell – triggers the alert.

2. Transmission: The Message Carrier

- Neural Pathways: Picture these signals racing like sprinters on a track, moving from your foot towards your brain. They're hurrying to deliver the message: "Something's wrong!"

- Pain Fibers: Some sprinters (A-delta fibres) are faster, telling your brain about sharp, immediate dangers. Others (C fibres) are slower, conveying a deep, lingering ache.

3. Processing: The Switchboard

- Spinal Reflexes: Before the sprinters even reach the brain, a local coach (the spinal cord) sees the problem and makes you instantly retract your foot. It's an immediate response, even before you consciously register the pain.

- Thalamus: When the signals do reach the brain, they first arrive at a bustling train station (the thalamus), which decides which tracks (brain areas) they should go to.

4. Perception: The Conscious Experience

- Cerebral Cortex: Here in the main hall of the brain, the message is translated into conscious thought: "Ouch! That shell was sharp!" This area discerns the type and quality of the pain, helping you understand it.

- Pain as a Multisensory Experience: Just as seeing the offending shell can heighten your reaction, past memories (like recalling a previous painful shell encounter) can influence your current perception.

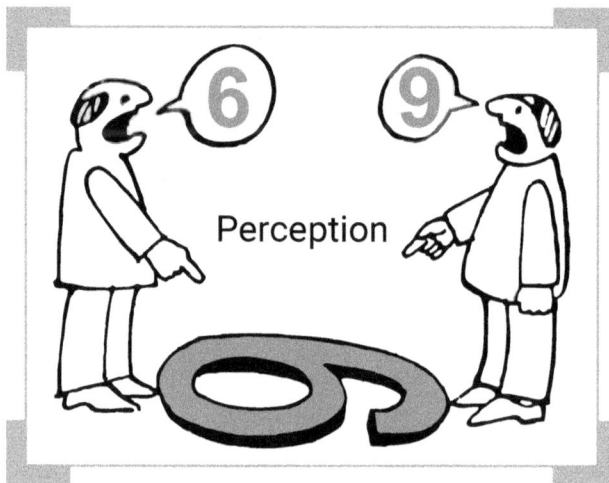

5. Emotional Response: The Heart of Pain

- Limbic System: Beyond just the physical sensation, there's an emotional theatre in your brain. Here, you might feel annoyance for not being more careful or a flash of anger at the unseen shell.

- Amplification or Attenuation: If you're already anxious about navigating the beach, the pain might feel worse. But if you're distracted by a beautiful sunset, the pain's edge might soften a bit.

6. Modulation: The Regulator

- Descending Pathways: From the brain's control tower, signals can be sent back down, perhaps to soothe the pain a bit, telling the foot, "It's okay, we've got this."

- Endogenous Pain Control: Sometimes, the brain releases its own special medicine (like endorphins), which act like a gentle balm, softening the sting of the pain.

Through this journey, from the sands of a beach to the grand halls of the brain, we see that pain is more than just a reaction. It's a story crafted from the inputs of our environment, our brains' interpretations, and our hearts' emotions.

3. THE UNSEEN GUARDIAN

In the quiet town of Gatineau,15-year-old Sophia always wore a golden bracelet, a family heirloom passed down for generations. Nobody knew, not even Sophia, that the bracelet possessed an unusual power: it could transform pain sensations.

One sunny day, as Sophia wandered the forest edge near her home, she tripped over an unseen root and felt her ankle twist. Ordinarily, such a misstep would result in sharp pain, but instead, she felt a gentle warmth envelop her ankle. A soft luminescence radiated from her bracelet, and the sensation moved up her arm and into her chest.

Confused, Sophia sat down and inspected her foot. It was unmistakably swollen, the telltale sign of a sprain. But instead of pain, she felt a series of sensations she couldn't describe, as if the forest around her was sharing its energy, wrapping her injury in a protective cocoon. The wind whispered comforting words, and the rustling leaves felt like the forest's lullaby.

As Sophia tried to comprehend this phenomenon, an elderly woman, known to the villagers as the sage Nana, approached her. With a knowing smile, she said, "Your bracelet, dear child, carries the power of our ancestors. It converts physical pain into sensations that can be borne more easily, connecting you with the world around to share its burden."

Sophia looked down at her bracelet, its glow now subdued. She realized that with every scrape and every bruise she had gotten as a child, the bracelet had protected her, turning potential pain into an experience she could understand and cope with.

Nana continued, "The bracelet doesn't eliminate injury but changes how you perceive it. It's a guardian, teaching you that pain, while real, can be experienced differently with a little help."

Sophia smiled, gratitude swelling in her heart for her unseen guardian. She thanked Nana and limped back home, feeling more connected to her ancestors and the world around her than ever before.

From that day on, Sophia's perspective on pain shifted. She learned that while pain is an inevitable part of life, our perception of it can be influenced, moulded, and sometimes, even transformed.

Key Message

This section emphasizes the pain journey from mere sensory input to a complex perception shaped by various internal and external factors. It underscores the need to approach pain as a symptom and a narrative of the body's experiences. Together, these subtitles and their respective elaborations offer a panoramic view of pain, encouraging readers to appreciate its complexities and the necessity for individualized, comprehensive approaches to its management.

Reflection Exercise:

Use the following questions as a guide for your reflection. Write your responses in the space provided or in a separate document.

1.   For Patients: How does understanding pain as both a sensory and emotional experience change the way you think about your pain, and how might this perspective influence your approach to managing it?

Response: _____

_____

_____

2.   For Providers: How can incorporating the IASP's emphasis on the emotional dimension of pain into your practice improve your treatment strategies, and how might this holistic understanding impact patient outcomes?

Response: _____

_____

_____

3.   In what ways does the story illustrate the idea that perception can influence the experience of pain? How can this concept be applied in your situations?

Response: _____

_____

_____

4. How does the forest setting and environment contribute to the overall mood and message of the story? What might the forest represent in Sophia's journey?

Response: _____

_____

_____

5. Reflect on a time in your own life when you experienced pain (physical or emotional). How did your perception of the pain affect your ability to cope with it?

Response: _____

_____

_____

True or False:

6. Pain is an illusion and doesn't need to be acknowledged.

7. Pain can be completely avoided with the right tools.

8. Pain is inevitable, but our perception of it can be transformed.

9. Pain should be ignored and never addressed directly.

Answers:

6. False

7. False

8. True

9. False

Idea:

By the end of the story, Sophia learns that pain is an inevitable part of life, but our perception of it can be transformed. Her magical bracelet does not eliminate pain but changes how she experiences it, turning it into more bearable sensations. This lesson teaches Sophia that while we cannot avoid pain, we can influence how we perceive and cope with it, making it easier to manage and understand. This concept is captured in option (6).

4. UNRAVELING THE EVOLUTIONS IN PERSISTENT PAIN PATHOPHYSIOLOGY: A CONTEMPORARY OVERVIEW

Research into persistent pain mechanisms is advancing, uncovering potential paths for targeted treatments. However, the complexity of these mechanisms and their vast interplay at cellular and subcellular levels complicate therapeutic approaches due to side effects. This review sheds light on four promising research areas: nerve growth factor antagonists, microglia's role in the CNS, AMPK activators, and genetic influences on pain perception.

The Mysterious Role of Microglia in the Tale of Neuropathic Pain

In the intricate maze of the Central Nervous System (CNS), microglia stand out as vigilant guardians. Born from embryonic mesoderm, they find their way to the CNS and craft and refine neuronal circuits for an entire lifetime. Within the hippocampus's deep corridors and the spinal cord's vast plains, these cells account for nearly 20% of all CNS inhabitants (Lema, 2020).

However, beneath their silent facade, they have a secret. These guardians hold a key to the puzzling world of neuropathic pain, a ghostly pain arising from nerve damage. Microglia awaken when a nerve suffers an injury, like a soldier sounding an alarm. This process, termed "microgliosis," propels them into action – from safeguarding the wounded nerves to summoning an army of inflammatory agents.

Amid this orchestrated response, the MAPK pathway emerges as the crucial player, a series of chemical messages that ignite the inflammation. The MAPK's roster includes potent entities like p38 protein and the formidable c-Jun N-terminal kinase. When provoked by forces like the notorious TNF-α or the omnipresent ATP, the microglia activate their p38 MAPK pathways. What follows is a cascade of events leading to increased pain signals, weakening the brain's natural defences against pain.

Amidst this chaos, a ray of hope gleams. Scientists discovered that minocycline, a humble antibiotic when introduced directly into the spinal fluid, could tame the fierce microglia and alleviate the agonizing pain. Meanwhile, innovations like spinal cord stimulation are being tested, aiming at the very regions enriched with these glial cells. The hope? To revolutionize pain management.

AMPK Activators: A New Hope

Another story unfolds around AMPK, an enzyme resembling a vigilant custodian of cellular energy. When a cell faces threats, AMPK springs into action to restore harmony. Interestingly, AMPK has the power to suppress the very pathways causing chronic pain, like the infamous MAPK (Lema, 2020).

Scientists have turned to compounds like metformin and O304 in their search for solutions. While metformin, a common anti-diabetic drug, activates AMPK indirectly, O304, a more refined player, specifically targets AMPK. When put to the test, these agents showed promising results in mouse models, kindling hopes of a brighter future for pain management.

The Genetic Web of Pain

While microglia and AMPK narrate their tales, a different story unravels at the genetic level. Our DNA hides clues about our pain experiences and susceptibilities. The genes responsible for drug metabolism, for instance, can determine how one responds to opioids. Because of their genetic makeup, some might find codeine utterly ineffective, while others might be overwhelmed by its effects.

Dopamine receptors, intricately linked with addiction, add another layer to the plot. Genetic variations in these receptors might predispose some to heroin addiction, painting a clear picture of the strong genetic underpinnings of substance dependence.

But the genetic tale of pain doesn't end there. Channelopathies, a group of disorders arising from defects in ion channel function, bring a slew of painful and painless conditions. Mutations in a single gene, like SCN9A, can either grant immunity to pain or lead to unbearable conditions like erythromelalgia (Lema, 2020).

Advancing Insights: The Nexus of Research and Innovation

As our knowledge expands, there's a move towards creating specialized societies for in-depth study on specific topics. Despite the significant growth in specialized understanding of chronic pain, a comprehensive approach is essential to keep patients at the forefront. "Frontiers in Pain Research" is well-positioned with its wide-ranging editorial board to support the holistic Pain 360 vision.

Dr. Hartrick mused on a pressing dilemma in a bustling research facility: the dire need for new pain-relief drugs and the hurdles in introducing fresh, innovative molecules into the medical market. As he navigated the labyrinthine corridors of drug discovery, he felt the potential locked away in understanding the body's own markers – the physiological changes that heralded pain and the biomarkers that might point towards its treatment. The idea of using actual human tissue outside the body as a preliminary testbed for these new drugs' effectiveness and safety seemed revolutionary, but it held promise.

Not far away, in another wing of a similar research facility, Dr. De Andres and his team were diving deep into the intricacies of the spine. Their focus was on a technique known as intrathecal drug delivery, a method to administer medication directly into the space around the spinal cord. They wielded state-of-the-art imaging tools, revealing details previously unseen and guiding them toward optimal device placements and dosages. But even with all this advanced tech, mysteries persisted. Dr. De Andres was particularly intrigued by the peridural membrane, an often-overlooked part of our anatomy. "There's more to it than meets the eye," he often remarked.

Meanwhile, in a room filled with computer screens showcasing fluid dynamic simulations, Bosscher was engrossed in mathematical models. His work sought to understand what happens when fluids are forcefully injected into the epidural space of the spine. The colourful simulations on his screens weren't just visually arresting; they held clues for vital safety protocols for future treatments.

In another research building dedicated to the mysteries of the brain, Robayo and her team were working with patients who had suffered traumatic brain injuries (TBI). They weren't just conducting routine tests but trying to decipher specific pain profiles and unique patterns that might pave the way for more tailored treatments. Robayo believed that by understanding these human-centric pain patterns, they might better tweak their animal models for research, circling back to the foundational concepts of pain understanding (Hartrick CT, 2023).

Research on the Nav1.7 channel, crucial to the nociception pathway, has revealed its potential as a target for pain management. Shields and his team identified inhibitors that showed promising antinociceptive properties. Although existing painkillers, like carbamazepine, provide relief, their broad action on multiple channels can limit effectiveness. There's an intriguing interplay between the Nav1.7 channel and the opioid system, suggesting a potential combined therapeutic approach. Furthermore, genes such as SCN9A and SCN11A have been pinpointed concerning pain perception. As scientists delve deeper, understanding the nuances of these pathways can revolutionize pain medical treatment strategies (Cascella, 2022).

Key message:

While working on diverse projects, all these researchers shared a common goal: to understand, confront, and hopefully alleviate the enigma of pain, making life better for countless individuals. The realm of neuropathic pain is vast and mysterious, with microglia, AMPK, and genetics weaving intertwining tales. As scientists and doctors strive to unravel these stories, one thing becomes clear: understanding these narratives is the key to conquering the world of pain.

Reflection Exercise:

Use the following questions as a guide for your reflection. Write your responses in the space provided or in a separate document. These questions are designed to foster a deeper understanding and engagement with ongoing research and its potential impact on patient care and treatment outcomes.

FOR PATIENTS:

1.   How does learning about the complex mechanisms of persistent pain affect your perception of your own pain experience?

Response: _____

_____

_____

2.   What are your thoughts on the idea that genetics can influence pain perception and the effectiveness of pain treatments?

Response: _____

_____

_____

3.   What has been your experience with current pain management strategies, including medication, physical therapy, or alternative therapies?

Response: _____

_____

_____

4.   Have you encountered any side effects from your current treatments that you find particularly challenging?

Response: _____

_____

_____

5.   What are your expectations or hopes from ongoing research into pain mechanisms and new treatments?

Response: _____

_____

_____

For Health Providers

1.   How do the recent advancements in understanding microglia's role in neuropathic pain influence your approach to patient care?

Response: _____

_____

_____

2.   How do you communicate complex scientific information about pain mechanisms and new treatments to your patients in an understandable way?

Response: _____

_____

_____

3.   What strategies do you use to manage patients' expectations regarding new and emerging pain treatments?

Response: _____

_____

_____

4. What role do multidisciplinary teams play in advancing pain management and incorporating new research findings into practice?

Response: _____

_____

_____

Idea: Recent research into persistent pain mechanisms is uncovering promising treatments despite the complexity of these mechanisms. Key areas of focus include nerve growth factor antagonists, the role of microglia in the CNS, AMPK activators, and genetic influences on pain perception. These advancements highlight the potential of targeting specific pain pathways and genetic factors to develop personalized pain management strategies.

5. AMELIA'S DANCE WITH SHADOWS: AN ODYSSEY THROUGH CHRONIC PAIN

Elmsworth, a town known for its picturesque landscapes and time-capsuled architecture, was home to Amelia in northern Alberta, Canada. Her quaint house, nestled amidst whispering willows and century-old oaks, had been part of her family lineage for generations. Each brick and tile whispered stories of the past, and just as the house bore the weight of history, Amelia carried an invisible weight of her own.

To the townsfolk, Amelia was a beacon of inspiration. Her laughter was infectious, echoing through Elmsworth's cobbled streets, filling hearts with joy. But beneath the façade of joviality, she bore the relentless burden of chronic pain, a relentless opponent that refused to back down.

Every sunrise brought hope but also a reminder of her daily combat. Mornings were deceptive, with the world painted in hues of oranges and purples. A soft, tingling sensation often greeted her, only to escalate into an agonizing crescendo by midday. To Amelia, it felt as though she was trapped in an opera where the notes grew increasingly out of tune, reaching a disharmonious climax.

Despite seeking remedies, Amelia often felt like a ship caught in a tempest with no land in sight. Each doctor's therapy was like a lighthouse, offering a glimmer of hope. But the storm of her pain consistently proved overwhelming, often leaving her lost at sea.

Yet, amid the tempestuous waves of anguish, Amelia sought solace in the little alcoves of life. She would often be found engrossed in books, travelling to distant lands through their pages, momentarily escaping the clutches of her ailment. The act of planting a seed in her garden and watching it grow became a symbolic defiance against her pain, life, growth, and beauty in the face of adversity.

One golden evening, while Amelia was engrossed in painting a scene from her favourite book by the riverbank, Lina approached her. Lina's gait, slightly staggered but determined, told a story strikingly similar to Amelia's. Their shared experience of pain was a language of its own — words weren't necessary. Lina introduced Amelia to the world of dance therapy, a medium that allowed them to channel their pain into graceful movements, turning their agony into an art form.

The duo's shared cathartic experiences gave birth to the idea of "Whispered Echoes." They envisioned it as a sanctuary where souls burdened by chronic pain could gather, share, heal, and find strength in unity. From meditation workshops to art sessions dance routines to storytelling evenings, they crafted a realm where pain could be acknowledged and transformed into powerful narratives.

Word spread and the once-small group expanded. The town's old community hall soon echoed with the resonating tales of resilience and hope. Amelia's house became a center of workshops, with every room humming with activity. The garden bloomed with flowers and the laughter of those who found strength in shared experiences.

Amelia's narrative became a guiding light for many. Through the darkest tunnels of her pain, she illuminated pathways for countless others, demonstrating that one could either be consumed by pain or harness it, turning it into a powerful force of transformation.

Her story reverberated across Elmsworth and beyond, inspiring many to dance, even with shadows, to find melodies in the cacophony, and to paint with all shades, dark and bright. Amelia's odyssey wasn't just about enduring pain but transforming it, making it a poignant part of a larger, beautiful canvas.

Reflection Exercise:

Use the following questions as a guide for your reflection. Write your responses in the space provided or in a separate document. These questions are designed to foster a deeper understanding and engagement with ongoing research and its potential impact on patient care and treatment outcomes.

FOR PATIENTS:

1. In what ways do you relate to Amelia's journey and experiences? Have you ever felt like you were battling an invisible opponent in your life?

Response: _____

_____

_____

2. How do you perceive Amelia's strength and resilience in the face of her chronic pain? Can you recall a time when you had to draw upon similar qualities?

Response: _____

_____

_____

3. Amelia finds solace in books, gardening, and, eventually, dance therapy. What are your personal methods for coping with difficult situations or chronic challenges?

Response: _____

_____

_____

4. Amelia turned her pain into a force for creating "Whispered Echoes." Have you ever transformed a difficult experience into something positive or helpful for others?

Response: _____

_____

_____

5. Despite her pain, Amelia found joy in painting and other activities. What passions would you like to pursue regardless of the challenges you face?

Response: _____

_____

_____

For Health Providers:

6. How do you encourage your patients to find and use coping strategies like those used by Amelia (e.g., art, gardening, dance therapy)?

Response: _____

_____

_____

7. What methods do you use to empower your patients to manage their health and pain actively?

Response: _____

_____

_____

8. How do you gather patient feedback about their treatment experiences, and how do you use this feedback to improve your practice?

Response: _____

_____

_____

Idea: The story of Amelia illustrates that sharing personal experiences can foster empathy and support, and engaging in joyful activities can help manage chronic pain. It underscores the importance of community, transforming pain into positive action, and pursuing passions despite challenges. This highlights the need for patient-centred care, effective communication, diverse support mechanisms, and collaboration among healthcare providers. Empowering patients and creating new support initiatives can enhance outcomes and build a holistic, empathetic healthcare environment.

6. SILENT BATTLES, LOUD COURAGE: CHRONICLES OF MEDICA'S UNSUNG HEROES

Amid the intertwining streets of Medica, each corner, every building, and every face tells a tale. The city pulsates with life yet beneath its lively exterior lie stories of perseverance and courage.

Osteoarthritis:

Martha's cozy home is filled with the gentle sound of piano melodies. Antique furniture and family portraits adorn her living room, but the most precious item is the old grand piano, a gift from her grandmother. Once, Martha's fingers danced effortlessly on the keys, bringing to life the compositions of Chopin and Beethoven. Each note celebrated her love for music and a testament to her talent. Now, every stiffened joint and painful stretch echo memories of recitals, joy, and passion. Despite her osteoarthritis, Martha refuses to give up. She adapts her playing style, finding new ways to express herself through the music she loves.

Rheumatoid Arthritis:

An IT specialist, Liam loves his morning jogs in Medica's central park. The fresh air and rhythmic pounding of his feet on the path are his sanctuary. Recently, he's been seen sporting wrist supports. His colleagues wonder why a young man wears them, not knowing that some mornings, Liam struggles even to type emails, his fingers betraying him with inflammation. The pain and stiffness in his joints are unpredictable, often making simple tasks daunting. Nevertheless, Liam approaches each day with determination, finding strength in routine and the support of his loved ones.

Fibromyalgia:

Sarah's apartment walls are lined with awards and newspaper clippings showcasing her achievements. As a renowned journalist, she has covered stories from the farthest corners of the globe, bringing light to untold tales. Yet, what isn't displayed is her battle with fibromyalgia. Her notebooks contain not just interview notes but also daily pain diaries, tracking the ebb and flow of discomfort. Each day is a challenge, as fatigue and widespread pain threaten to overwhelm her. Still, Sarah perseveres, using her platform to raise awareness about her condition, hoping to inspire others who face similar battles.

Chronic Back Pain:

John's little daughter often asks why he grimaces when he lifts her. The walls of their home are filled with photos of skyscrapers and monuments to John's years of labour in construction. Each building stands tall, a symbol of his hard work and dedication. But each brick and girder also speaks of the toll taken on his back. Chronic back pain is a constant companion, making even the simplest movements a struggle. Despite the pain, John's love for his daughter and his passion for building keeps him going. He dreams of the day when he can lift her without wincing and works tirelessly to find relief.

Neuropathic Pain:

Miguel's dance studio, 'Flaming Feet,' is the talk of Medica. The studio is a vibrant space filled with energy and rhythm where students of all ages come to learn the art of dance. Miguel often takes breaks while his students dance with abandon, massaging his feet and reminiscing about his days in Seville before neuropathy's fiery steps joined his dance. The burning pain in his feet is relentless, starkly contrasting to the graceful movements he once performed easily. Yet, Miguel remains a passionate teacher, inspiring his students with his resilience and dedication to the art of dance.

Migraines:

Fatima's quaint corner in Medica's library is an oasis of calm. Surrounded by towering shelves of books, she finds solace in the written word. But there's a drawer filled with migraine medications, sunglasses, and earplugs. On stormy days, when migraines loom, she retreats into her sanctuary, dimming lights and seeking refuge among silent books. The throbbing pain and sensitivity to light and sound can be debilitating, but Fatima's love for literature helps her endure. She uses her experience to curate special reading lists for others with chronic pain, offering them a similar escape.

TMJ Disorders:

At the 'Medica Melodies' opera house, Clara's voice resonates with emotion, captivating audiences with its power and beauty. However, backstage, she's often seen with a cold pack, easing the pain accompanying her high notes. Temporomandibular joint (TMJ) disorders have made singing a painful endeavour, each performance a test of endurance. Despite the challenges, Clara's passion for music and determination to perform drive her forward. She works closely with vocal coaches and therapists, finding ways to manage her pain and continue sharing her gift with the world.

Chronic Fatigue Syndrome:

Leo's athletic achievements adorn the 'Medica Sports Hall.' Trophies and medals tell the story of a once unstoppable athlete who dominated every field. Yet, Leo now champions a different cause: Chronic Fatigue

Syndrome (CFS) awareness. His new marathon is to educate Medica about the fatigue that binds his once tireless legs. The constant exhaustion and unrefreshing sleep are invisible weights he carries daily. Leo's advocacy work aims to shed light on CFS, offering support and understanding to others who struggle with this misunderstood condition.

Irritable Bowel Syndrome:

Naomi's restaurant, 'Gastronomic Delights,' is a culinary haven known for its innovative dishes and welcoming atmosphere. She experiments with recipes to cater to those with Irritable Bowel Syndrome (IBS), turning her personal challenges into gastronomic innovations. Each menu item is crafted with care, balancing flavours and ingredients to ensure they are both delicious and gentle on the digestive system. Naomi's journey with IBS has inspired her to create a space where others with similar dietary needs can enjoy gourmet meals without fear.

Complex Regional Pain Syndrome:

Jake's fire station showcases medals of bravery, each one a testament to his courage and dedication. But there's one flame he battles privately: the burning sensation in his leg caused by Complex Regional Pain Syndrome (CRPS). The pain is unrelenting, a constant reminder of his injury. His new mission is finding relief, ensuring the fire within doesn't consume his spirit. Jake's strength and determination are evident as he continues to serve his community, inspiring his fellow firefighters with his resilience and commitment.

Post-surgical Pain:

Rosa's garden blooms with vibrant roses, each one a symbol of beauty and resilience. Each rose, though beautiful, reminds her of the surgical scars and persistent pain she endures. The garden is her sanctuary, a place where she can find peace and solace amidst the flowers. Despite the pain, Rosa's green thumb and her passion for gardening help her cope. She finds joy in nurturing her plants, each new bloom a testament to her strength and hope amidst adversity.

In Medica, stories of chronic pain merge into a mosaic of resilience, illustrating the indomitable spirit of its citizens. Each individual's journey is a testament to their courage and determination, transforming silent battles into loud courage.

Key Message:

Chronic pain, regardless of its specific diagnosis, often presents with similar challenges and experiences across different conditions. Individuals with chronic pain, whether from osteoarthritis, rheumatoid arthritis, fibromyalgia, chronic back pain, neuropathic pain, migraines, TMJ disorders, chronic fatigue syndrome, irritable bowel syndrome, complex regional pain syndrome, or post-surgical pain, face a daily battle that goes beyond physical symptoms. Common threads include persistent and often debilitating pain, fatigue, emotional distress, and a significant impact on quality of life. These conditions may differ in their specific triggers and manifestations, but they universally require individuals to find ways to manage pain, seek effective treatments, and maintain hope and resilience. The stories of Medica's citizens illustrate that despite the different labels of their diagnoses, the core experience of chronic pain unites them in their struggle and strength, highlighting the need for empathetic and holistic approaches in healthcare.

Reflection Exercise:

Use the following questions as a guide for your reflection. Write your responses in the space provided or in a separate document. These reflective questions are designed to explore the impact of specific diagnosis labels on the experience and management of chronic pain, encouraging deeper understanding and empathy in both patients and health providers.

FOR PATIENTS:

1. Which story from Medica resonates the most with your own experience? Why?

Response: _____

_____

_____

2. How has your condition affected your ability to engage in activities you once enjoyed, similar to Martha's experience with her piano playing?

Response: _____

_____

_____

3. Have you found ways to turn your pain into something positive, as Naomi did with her restaurant or Leo with his advocacy work?

Response: _____

_____

_____

FOR HEALTH PROVIDERS:

4. How do you recognize and address the common threads of chronic pain, such as persistent pain, fatigue, and emotional distress, in your patients?

Response: _____

_____

_____

5. How do you consider the specific diagnosis labels (e.g., rheumatoid arthritis, migraines) when developing treatment plans for patients with chronic pain? Do these labels significantly influence your approach?

Response: _____

_____

_____

6. How do you address the potential biases or misconceptions that might arise from specific diagnosis labels when treating patients with chronic pain?

Response: _____

_____

_____

True or False Questions

1. Chronic pain conditions often present with similar challenges and experiences, regardless of the specific diagnosis.

2. Osteoarthritis only affects the elderly and is not seen in younger individuals.

3. Emotional distress is a common thread among individuals with different chronic pain conditions.

4. The specific label of a chronic pain diagnosis does not influence the treatment approach by healthcare providers.

5. All chronic pain conditions have clear and predictable triggers.

6. Patients with chronic pain often need to adapt their daily activities to manage their symptoms.

7. A diagnosis label like fibromyalgia or rheumatoid arthritis can affect how patients are perceived and treated by others.

8. Patients with chronic pain should not be encouraged to participate in activities they enjoy due to the risk of exacerbating their condition.

Answers

1. True

2. False

3. True

4. False

5. False

6. True

7. True

8. False

Idea: Chronic pain, despite varying diagnoses, presents similar challenges like persistent pain, fatigue, and emotional distress. Effective management includes medical treatments and holistic approaches such as art therapy. Community and peer support and empathy from healthcare providers are crucial for patient care. Diagnosis labels influence treatment and perception, but sharing coping strategies across conditions is beneficial. Encouraging enjoyable activities fosters resilience and well-being.

THE VICIOUS CYCLE OF CHRONIC PAIN AND PSYCHOLOGY

*"The body always leads us to the truth, but it's
the mind that decides if we follow."*
Deepak Chopra

Synopses: In this chapter, we delve into the intricate relationship between chronic pain and psychology. Chronic pain isn't just a physical sensation; it has profound psychological effects, influencing emotions, behaviours, and overall mental health. Similarly, a person's psychological state can intensify pain perception, creating a cyclical pattern that's challenging to break. We'll explore how chronic pain can lead to psychological distress, including anxiety, depression, and cognitive changes. Conversely, we'll discuss how one's mental state can amplify pain sensations, perpetuating the cycle. Understanding this interplay is crucial for holistic pain management strategies, which this chapter seeks to illuminate. Readers will gain insight into the complexities of pain, its psychosocial impacts, and potential therapeutic approaches that address physical and psychological facets.

The role of psychology in understanding and treating pain has been acknowledged since early theories of nociception. These theories recognized the influence of midbrain and cortical structures in pain expression. In the 1950s and 1960s, the psychology of behaviour expanded, highlighting the role of the environment in shaping treatment and complaining behaviour related to pain. These clinical theories emerged due to the challenges posed by chronic pain and disability in patients. Psychology became integral to pain treatments as it became evident that many patients reported levels of complaint and disability that couldn't be solely explained by the extent of damage or disease (Eccleston, 2001).

When discussing chronic pain, it's important to realize that the emotional and cognitive response to persistent pain often forms a feedback loop, with each element influencing and amplifying the other.

Feelings of sadness, anxiety, or anger can intensify the experience of pain. Pain experiences, when coupled with intense negative emotions, can be perceived as more severe than they might be in a neutral emotional state. Thoughts such as "This pain will never end" or "I can't do anything right because of my pain" can trap individuals in a pessimistic mindset. Such distorted beliefs can exacerbate the emotional distress tied to the pain, thereby increasing its perceived intensity.

Psychological treatments play a vital role in the multidisciplinary management of chronic pain. They aid in enhancing pain self-management, strengthening pain-coping strategies, decreasing pain-related disability, and minimizing emotional distress. Through various self-regulatory, behavioural, and cognitive methods, psychologists help patients regain control over their pain, leading to a more normal life. These interventions equip patients with skills, making them proactive in their illness management and providing lifelong benefits. An integrated approach to chronic pain also promotes returning to work, cuts healthcare costs, and improves the health-related quality of life for countless global patients (Roditi & Robinson, 2011)

In the crazy maze of dealing with chronic pain, there's this cool, less-talked-about tool: psychology. Imagine wielding the power to manage pain better, dial down the emotional rollercoaster, and chop down disability linked to pain. That's what psychological strategies bring to the table. They're like a personal trainer for your brain, prepping it to fight pain. And here's the kicker: not only do patients get better at handling their current pain, but they also pick up these rockstar skills that serve them for life.

What's more? Toss in the perks of potentially getting back to the daily grind faster, saving some serious cash on health bills, and boosting the overall vibe of life. Millions of people worldwide can tap into these benefits. Chronic pain management isn't just meds and therapy; it's a mindset game, too!

THE COGNITIVE IMPACT OF CHRONIC PAIN

The increasing prevalence of pain-related conditions has intensified research into understanding the neurological bases of pain and its effects on cognition. Various studies indicate disruptions in cognitive processes across numerous chronic pain conditions. While the precise mechanisms remain elusive, one theory posits that chronic pain might strain the brain's resources, leading to cognitive deficits. This is further supported by preclinical research on rodents, though such studies are limited despite the existence of validated animal models (Moriarty, McGuire, & Finn, 2011).

Animal models have revealed pain-related alterations in brain structures. Specifically, research by Seminowicz et al. (2009) identified significant volume decreases in specific brain regions of rats subjected to pain, suggesting structural changes could correlate with pain perception. In terms of treatment, addressing chronic pain remains challenging. Current strategies predominantly target the sensory components of pain with medications like NSAIDs.

There's a consensus across both preclinical and clinical studies linking pain to cognitive impairments. These deficits can substantially affect daily tasks, deteriorating the quality of life for pain patients. Preliminary evidence also hints at a neuropathological basis for these cognitive disruptions (Moriarty, McGuire, & Finn, 2011).

ATTENTIONAL BIAS AND CHRONIC PAIN

Individuals with chronic pain might develop a heightened sensitivity or focus on pain-related cues. This constant vigilance can be mentally exhausting and might lead to decreased attention span for other tasks. Attentional bias refers to the tendency of our attention to be drawn more rapidly or intensely to specific stimuli over others. In the context of chronic pain patients, it signifies the heightened focus or sensitivity these patients have towards pain-related stimuli, often to the detriment of other stimuli. This chapter delves into the intricacies of attentional bias in chronic pain patients, its underlying mechanisms, and the implications for treatment.

Threatening pain captures attention and can lead to a focus on both the pain source and potential ways to escape or alleviate it. Some individuals have an elevated sensitivity to pain sensation, and in cases where pain is persistent or recurrent, a pattern of constant vigilance toward pain can develop. This vigilance to pain has been linked to higher pain intensity, increased use of healthcare services, and greater emotional distress in chronic low back pain patients. It also significantly predicts disability, distress, and healthcare resource utilization. Excessive attention to threat or hypervigilance may explain the observed anxiety and concentration difficulties in patients with conditions like diffuse idiopathic pain or fibromyalgia. Studies have shown that patients with fibromyalgia may have a lower pain threshold and higher pain tolerance compared to those with rheumatoid arthritis or non-pain control samples. Additionally, research has found that patients who frequently attend to diffuse bodily sensations are more vulnerable to interruptions by high-intensity pain, and this heightened and habitual attention to pain and bodily sensations is associated with higher levels of disability and distress in patients with chronic pain (Eccleston, 2001).

The human brain is inherently trained to prioritize stimuli that might signify threat or harm. For chronic pain patients, pain-related stimuli serve as constant reminders of their discomfort or potential harm. Over time, repeated exposure to pain can result in a kind of 'sensitization' where even minor pain-related cues can trigger a heightened response. Chronic pain patients might develop cognitive schemas where they expect pain in specific situations, leading them to focus more on pain-related cues.

Implications of attentional bias in chronic pain patients encompass disruptions in daily activities due to increased focus on pain, leading to decreased productivity and life quality. This constant focus can also heighten emotional disturbances, such as anxiety and depression. Additionally, the continual attention to pain might intensify its perceived severity, making it seem worse than it actually is.

Researchers use various tools and methods to measure attentional bias, like the dot-probe task or the Stroop test. Participants often respond more rapidly to pain-related words or images in these tasks, highlighting their bias. This provides valuable insights into the intensity of the bias and can inform therapeutic interventions.

Addressing attentional bias in treatment is crucial. Therapeutic interventions include Cognitive Behavioral Therapy (CBT) to help patients recognize and counteract pain-focused thoughts, mindfulness and meditation to center attention on the present, and Attentional Bias Modification, which uses computerized tasks to redirect attention away from pain-related cues.

Attentional bias in chronic pain patients underscores the intricate relationship between perception, attention, and pain. Recognizing and addressing this bias can play a pivotal role in managing chronic pain and improving the overall well-being of those afflicted. Future research and treatment modalities must consider this interplay for more holistic and effective patient care.

Todd and his colleagues' study published in 2023 is the first to explore whether changes in attentional bias predict daily pain interference beyond pain severity. The study identifies factors like readiness to acquire attentional bias and resistance to change as necessary. Using a daily pain diary for more accurate data, the study sheds light on how attentional bias malleability can mitigate pain interference. Future research may refine attentional bias modification techniques to improve pain prevention and management strategies. (Todd, Clarke, Hughes, & van Ryckeghem, 2023)

MEMORY IMPAIRMENTS AND CHRONIC PAIN

Chronic pain, defined as persistent discomfort extending beyond the usual recovery period, not only affects physical health but also profoundly influences cognitive functions, particularly memory. This chapter delves deep into the relationship between chronic pain and memory impairments, exploring underlying mechanisms and the implications for patients with chronic pain that can affect cognitive processes like memory. People might find it hard to recall times when they were pain-free or might obsessively remember instances when the pain was especially severe. Chronic pain and memory are interconnected through intricate neural pathways. Chronic pain can cause structural and functional changes in the brain, especially in memory-related areas like the hippocampus. It also increases stress, leading to higher cortisol levels and adversely affecting memory.

Additionally, the attention required to manage chronic pain can limit cognitive resources essential for consolidating memories. Study on older community residents over an extended period indicates that those with chronic pain experience greater cognitive decline, especially in processing speed. This decline occurs regardless of factors like depression, opioid use, or other health issues. Therefore, it's crucial to treat chronic pain using both drug-based and non-drug strategies to prevent related cognitive effects (Rouch, et al., 2023).

Chronic pain can influence various aspects of memory:

- Short-term Memory: Patients may find retaining or recalling recently learned information challenging.

- Long-term Memory: Chronic pain might hinder the consolidation of memories or the ability to retrieve them effectively.

- Working Memory: The capacity to hold and manipulate information over short periods can be compromised, affecting tasks such as calculations or reading comprehension.

3. Impact on Daily Life

Memory impairments can drastically affect the daily lives of chronic pain patients:

- Decreased Productivity: Challenges in memory can hinder work performance and lead to increased mistakes.

- Social Implications: Forgetfulness might strain personal relationships or lead to social isolation.

- Self-care Challenges: Forgetting medications or therapy sessions can hinder effective pain management.

Memory impairment in chronic pain patients is substantial, but the aspects of memory (e.g. working memory, long-term memory, and autobiographical memory) in chronic pain patients and the potentially related factors (e.g. age, level of education, pain conditions, emotion, neural network, and use of analgesics) are modest. Memory impairment is interpreted with attention-narrowing and capacity-reduction hypotheses (Liu X, 2014).

APPROACHES TO MITIGATE MEMORY IMPAIRMENT

Recognizing the link between chronic pain and memory loss highlights the need for interventions. These include cognitive training exercises, effective pain management, and lifestyle changes such as proper sleep, nutrition, and mindfulness to support memory health in the presence of chronic pain.

The link between chronic pain and memory impairment is evident, but there are still complexities to unravel. Thorough research is needed to understand this complex relationship better and develop personalized therapeutic strategies. Embracing advancements, like neuroimaging, can significantly aid in comprehending and addressing these impairments.

Chronic pain is more than just physical suffering; it significantly impacts cognitive aspects, particularly memory. Acknowledging and mitigating these cognitive effects is crucial to improving patient well-being. This holistic perspective on chronic pain management is the future, and continued research offers hope for deeper understanding and innovative treatments.

BEHAVIOURAL RESPONSES AND THEIR IMPLICATIONS

Chronic pain influences more than just our physical well-being; it also deeply shapes our behaviours. Many behavioural patterns arise as a result of enduring pain, bringing substantial consequences for those affected. These behavioural responses can profoundly alter a person's daily life, overall wellness, and the trajectory of their pain journey. Let's delve deeper into some of these behavioural patterns and understand their implications.

1. Avoidance Behavior:

 - Description: Patients may avoid physical activity or situations that they believe will exacerbate their pain.

 - Implications: While avoidance might provide short-term relief, in the long run, it can lead to muscle atrophy, decreased physical fitness, increased disability, and social isolation. This can further reinforce the pain experience.

2. Pain Catastrophizing:

 - Description: This refers to negative cognitive and emotional processes where the individual magnifies the threat value of pain stimuli and feels helpless.

 - Implications: Catastrophizing is linked to higher pain intensity, increased emotional distress, and decreased pain tolerance. It can lead to increased utilization of healthcare resources without effective pain relief.

3. Excessive Rest:

 - Description: Believing that rest will help alleviate pain, some patients might rest more than necessary.

 - Implications: Excessive rest can lead to stiffness and muscle weakness and can exacerbate certain types of pain, such as fibromyalgia. It also impacts the person's ability to engage in daily activities, potentially leading to feelings of uselessness or depression.

4. Overactivity:

 - Description: In contrast to avoidance, some individuals push through the pain, ignoring their limits.

 - Implications: This can result in a "boom and bust" pattern where a person overexerts on "good days" and crashes on subsequent days. This inconsistent activity can increase pain and fatigue, making pain management even more challenging.

5. Pain Behaviors:

 - Description: Observable behaviours like limping, grimacing, or verbalizing about pain.

 - Implications: These behaviours can influence how others react to the individual. For instance, family members might become overly solicitous, reinforcing the pain behaviour. On the other hand, some might interpret the behaviours as attention-seeking, leading to potential invalidation of the pain experience.

6. Medication Overuse:

 - Description: Relying heavily on pain medications, sometimes even overusing them in an attempt to manage pain.

 - Implications: Overuse can lead to potential side effects, increased tolerance (needing more medication for the same effect), dependence, or even overdose. Additionally, it might mask the pain rather than address the root cause.

7. Emotional Responses:

 - Description: Chronic pain often comes with emotional reactions like depression, anxiety, anger, or frustration.

 - Implications: These emotional states can amplify the pain experience, creating a vicious cycle. They can also affect interpersonal relationships and reduce the effectiveness of pain management strategies.

8. Cognitive Impacts:

 - Description: Pain can affect cognitive functions like memory, attention, and decision-making.

 - Implications: This can further impair daily functioning, reduce work productivity, and affect interpersonal relationships. It might also reduce the patient's capacity to adhere to pain management regimens.

Behavioural responses to chronic pain can be as diverse as the pain experiences themselves. Recognizing these patterns and their potential implications is crucial in devising a comprehensive and effective pain management strategy. Both patients and healthcare providers must be aware of these behaviours and address them holistically.

Here's the deal: our reactions to chronic pain can be as varied as the ways we experience that pain. Spotting these behavioural twists and turns is key to creating a game plan that genuinely tackles the pain. For everyone in the pain journey – whether you're living with it or treating it – it's a must to understand and zoom in on these behaviours. And for the pros out there, knowing this inside out helps craft a plan that's tailored just right. We're talking about mixing things up – think cognitive-behavioural therapy (CBT), hands-on physical therapy, taking things step by step, some mindfulness meditation, and even meds when needed. Is it all about striking a balance between the body and mind and that combo? It can be a game-changer for those in pain.

THE SOCIAL RAMIFICATIONS OF LIVING WITH CHRONIC PAIN

Chronic pain, often an invisible ailment, has profound effects that permeate beyond the physical body. Among these ripple effects, the social consequences experienced by those suffering from chronic pain are particularly significant. This chapter delves into the multi-layered social implications of living with persistent pain, seeking to shed light on the challenges and the coping mechanisms employed by many.

1. Interpersonal Relationships and Familial Dynamics

Chronic pain doesn't only affect the individual but also the immediate circle around them.

- Misunderstandings and Misconceptions: Because chronic pain is often invisible, sufferers might encounter skepticism or lack of understanding from friends and family.

- Caregiver Fatigue: Loved ones who play a caregiving role can experience exhaustion, both emotionally and physically, as they continually support the pain sufferer.

- Shift in Roles: Established roles within a family or relationship might shift, with some members taking on more responsibilities to compensate.

2. Social Isolation and Withdrawal

For many, chronic pain can create barriers to social participation.

- Avoiding Social Gatherings: Pain flare-ups or the fear of them can deter individuals from attending gatherings, even if they wish to.

- Misunderstood Absences: Repeated cancellations can be misconstrued as disinterest, leading to strained friendships.

- Loneliness: The combination of physical pain and social isolation can culminate in feelings of loneliness, even when surrounded by loved ones.

3. Professional Impacts:

The workplace is another arena where the implications of chronic pain manifest.

- Decreased Productivity: Pain can impede concentration and task completion, leading to reduced output.

- Career Alterations: Some might need to change roles, reduce hours, or even retire earlier than intended due to their pain.

- Misjudgments at Work: Colleagues or superiors might misinterpret pain-induced fatigue or absences, potentially affecting professional relationships and growth.

4. The Struggle for Validation

One of the most profound social challenges faced by chronic pain sufferers is the quest for validation.

- Medical Gaslighting: Patients might encounter skepticism from medical professionals, feeling their pain is minimized or dismissed.

- Public Stigma: Misconceptions about chronic pain, especially when pain medication is involved, can result in judgments and biases from the broader society.

5. Building Resilient Communities

Despite the challenges, many find solace and strength in communities.

-Support Groups: Joining or creating support groups can provide an empathetic space for sharing experiences and coping strategies.

- Raising Awareness: Engaging in advocacy or awareness campaigns can create a broader societal understanding of chronic pain and its implications.

A recent study provides important new findings regarding the associations between social factors and the physical and psychological functioning of individuals with chronic pain, supporting biopsychosocial models (Solé, et al., 2022). Living with chronic pain is a journey fraught with social hurdles. However, understanding these challenges offers a pathway to empathy, support, and, ultimately, societal change. As we deepen our comprehension of the social ramifications of chronic pain, we're reminded of the resilience of the human spirit and the power of community.

THERAPEUTIC APPROACHES ADDRESSING PSYCHOLOGICAL DIMENSIONS

Chronic pain is not just a physical phenomenon; it also casts deep psychological shadows. To address the entirety of a patient's experience with pain, the medical community recognizes the importance of therapeutic interventions that target the psychological dimensions of pain. This chapter provides an overview of the most effective therapeutic approaches to address the emotional, cognitive, and psychological impacts of chronic pain.

1. Cognitive Behavioral Therapy (CBT)

At its core, CBT is a form of talk therapy that emphasizes the identification and restructuring of negative thought patterns and behaviours. It helps patients recognize and challenge pain-related negative thoughts, teaching strategies to cope more effectively. The patients often report decreased pain intensity, improved mood, and better functionality.

2. Mindfulness and Meditation

Embracing the Present: These practices focus on grounding individuals in the present moment, fostering a non-judgmental awareness of one's sensations and feelings. By being attuned to the present, patients can dissociate from their pain, viewing it as a sensation rather than a dominating experience. Regular practice can lead to reduced pain perception, enhanced relaxation, and better emotional regulation.

3. Acceptance and Commitment Therapy (ACT)

ACT, an offshoot of CBT, encourages acceptance of the pain while committing to values-driven actions. Instead of combating or avoiding pain, ACT teaches the embrace of pain as a part of the lived experience, redirecting energy toward meaningful activities. Patients often experience an enriched quality of life, a sense of purpose, and reduced distress.

4. Biofeedback and Relaxation Techniques

Tuning into the Body: These techniques involve gaining awareness of physiological functions to control and manage them. Patients learn to alter their physiological responses (like muscle tension) that exacerbate pain. Over time, patients can experience reduced pain levels and a greater sense of control over their bodies.

5. Group Therapy and Support Groups

The Power of Shared Experience: Being in a group setting allows individuals to share experiences, coping strategies, and support. Group settings, facilitated by a therapist or peer-led, allow for the communal exploration of pain challenges and victories. The feeling of being understood and the shared camaraderie can significantly uplift spirits and provide practical coping techniques.

6. Art and Music Therapy

Expressive Healing: These therapies use the mediums of art and music to allow individuals to express and process their experiences. By engaging in creative activities, patients can often articulate their pain experiences in ways words cannot capture. Many find relief in self-expression, reduced feelings of isolation, and an overall improvement in mood.

Addressing the psychological dimensions of chronic pain is as vital as managing its physical aspects. By integrating a holistic approach, therapeutic interventions can offer patients a fuller, more balanced path to coping and healing. Through these strategies, individuals can reclaim agency over their lives, transcending pain's limitations to find joy, purpose, and connection.

Key Message

Psychology plays a crucial role in understanding and treating chronic pain by addressing the emotional, cognitive, and behavioural aspects that influence pain perception and management. Psychological treatments enhance pain self-management, reduce pain-related disability, and decrease emotional distress, ultimately improving patients' quality of life and promoting a holistic approach to chronic pain management. Through strategies like cognitive-behavioral therapy, mindfulness, and acceptance and commitment therapy, patients can develop lifelong skills to manage pain effectively, leading to better health outcomes and lower healthcare costs.

Reflection Exercise

Use the following questions as a guide for your reflection. Write your responses in the space provided or in a separate document. These questions can foster deeper understanding and collaboration between patients and health providers, ultimately leading to more effective chronic pain management.

FOR PATIENTS:

1. Have you noticed any patterns in your thoughts and emotions that seem to amplify your pain?

Response: _____

_____

_____

2. Do you find yourself avoiding certain activities or social interactions because of your pain?

Response: _____

_____

_____

3. Have you communicated your pain experience to those around you, and how have they responded?

Response: _____

_____

_____

4. In what ways have your behaviours changed since experiencing chronic pain?

Response: _____

_____

_____

5. What negative thoughts or beliefs do you have about your pain and its impact on your life?

Response: _____

_____

_____

6. What goals do you have for improving your life despite the pain?

Response: _____

_____

_____

FOR HEALTH PROVIDERS:

7. How do you assess the psychological and emotional aspects of a patient's chronic pain?

Response: _____

_____

_____

8. What tools or techniques do you use to help patients redirect their focus away from pain-related cues?

Response: _____

_____

_____

9. How do you educate patients about the interplay between pain, emotions, and behaviours?

Response: _____

_____

_____

10. How do you ensure open and empathetic communication with patients about their pain experiences?

Response: _____

_____

_____

Idea: Chronic pain affects daily life and relationships, causing emotional distress and behavioural changes, like avoiding activities and social interactions, which lead to isolation. Memory and attention are often impaired, and negative thoughts worsen hopelessness. Effective coping strategies include mindfulness and gentle exercise, with psychological treatments being crucial. Open communication with loved ones is essential. *As a healthcare provider, I use interviews, questionnaires, and tools to assess pain's psychological aspects, integrating CBT, MBSR, and ACT into treatment. I educate patients on the connection between pain, emotions, and behaviours, recommending support groups. A holistic approach, combining psychological treatments with physical therapy, medication, and lifestyle changes, improves quality of life and daily functioning.*

ENTWINED: THE DANCE OF PAIN AND PSYCHE

Lana always thought the pain was straightforward. She'd experienced her fair share of it— from stubbing a toe to experiencing heartbreak— but none of that prepared her for the car accident she faced in her mid-20s. The incident was minor, but the resulting pain in her back wasn't. Days turned into weeks, weeks into months, and soon, Lana found herself in the throes of chronic pain.

She met Dr. Carter, a renowned psychologist, on a rainy Thursday afternoon. "Physical pain, Lana, has a way of weaving itself into the fabric of our psyche," he began after she narrated her ordeal.

The days were bearable, but nights were an endless loop of tossing and turning. The pain had now etched its presence not just on her back but also in her mind. The hurt from the accident began to meld with anxieties from her past, amplifying her physical discomfort.

A memory of a forgotten breakup or a childhood trauma would make her pain flare up. Conversely, on days the pain was too unbearable, memories of the accident and other past traumas seemed more vivid, almost cinematic.

Dr. Carter said, "Think of your pain and mind as two dancers, Lana. They move in tandem, feeding off each other's energy. If one falters, it's hard for the other to continue gracefully."

Lana soon realized that she wasn't only fighting against her backache. She was battling fears from her past and the accident's trauma that had settled deep within her.

Dr. Carter introduced her to various therapies that didn't just target the physical pain but also the mental scars she carried. Meditation, cognitive behavioural therapy, and even joining support groups became a part of her recovery regimen.

It was during one of these support group meetings that Lana met Michael. He had a similar story, stemming from a hiking accident. The two connected on shared experiences, providing solace and understanding to each other.

They began to share coping mechanisms. Michael introduced Lana to journaling while she showed him the calming world of watercolour painting. Together, they embarked on a journey to untangle the complex web of physical and psychological pain.

Over time, with consistent therapy and each other's support, the intensity of their chronic pain diminished. It never vanished entirely, but they learned to keep the psychological triggers at bay, ensuring the dance between pain and mind was more harmonious.

The story ended on a hopeful note for both. They realized that pain, whether physical or psychological, was an ever-present reality. Yet, understanding its intricate relationship and mastering its rhythm could lead to a semblance of peace.

Reflection Exercise:

1. How does Lana's journey with chronic pain following her car accident resonate with your own experiences of injury or trauma?

Response: _____

_____

_____

2. Have you noticed any specific memories or past traumas similar to Lana's that seem to amplify your physical pain?

Response: _____

_____

_____

3. How do you manage the interplay between your physical pain and mental health, as Lana did with her anxieties from the past?

Response: _____

_____

_____

4. Which therapies introduced by Dr. Carter, such as meditation and cognitive behavioural therapy, do you find most intriguing or relevant to your situation?

Response: _____

_____

_____

5. How do you think combining physical and psychological treatments can benefit your pain management, as it did for Lana?

Response: _____

_____

_____

6. What lessons can you take from Lana's journey about resilience and adapting to chronic pain?

Response: _____

_____

_____

Idea: Reflect on how your pain is connected to past traumas and emotions, like Lana's. Identify effective strategies, such as meditation and therapy, and recognize the importance of mutual support in managing pain. Embrace combining physical and psychological treatments, as Dr. Carter did for Lana, to enhance pain management. Draw lessons from Lana's resilience and set goals to incorporate these strategies into your daily routine for a balanced and harmonious life.

CHAPTER 5

THE SYNERGY OF PHYSICAL THERAPY & PSYCHOLOGICAL UNDERSTANDING: A STRATEGIC OVERVIEW

"Healing is not just about fixing the body; it's about understanding the mind. The synergy of physical and psychological therapies is essential."

Synopsis: Physical therapy, traditionally known for its biomechanical focus on body movements, function, and structure, has experienced a paradigm shift. Modern healthcare emphasizes the intertwining nature of the physical and psychological realms. This chapter seeks to illuminate the synergy between physical therapy and psychological understanding, showcasing how this integration can foster enhanced therapeutic outcomes.

Historically, physical therapy and psychology have been perceived as distinct domains. While physical therapists worked on the body's ailments, psychologists delved into the intricacies of the mind. However, as we've evolved in our understanding of holistic health, the boundary between these two fields has blurred, leading to the realization that optimal therapeutic outcomes hinge on their convergence.

Every physical ailment carries a psychological component. For instance, a patient with chronic pain might develop anxiety or depression. Similarly, a patient battling depression may neglect physical activity, leading to muscular atrophy or joint issues. Recognizing these intertwined effects can result in more effective and holistic interventions.

Chronic pain is a complex, multifaceted condition that often requires more than just traditional physical interventions to manage effectively— integrating psychological approaches into physical therapy (often referred to as psychologically informed physical therapy or PIPT) can be highly beneficial in addressing the multidimensional nature of chronic pain.

Emanuel Brunner, a physiotherapist at Kantonsspital Winterthur in Switzerland, specializes in treating patients with severe pain and conducts research at the University of Leuven in Belgium. His work emphasizes integrating psychological methods into physiotherapy for chronic musculoskeletal pain. His studies reveal that physiotherapists often misjudge psychological factors in patients with chronic low back pain and lack confidence in treating such cases. The research highlights a need for physiotherapists to receive more training in psychological aspects, as this patient demographic is expected to persist.

Psychologically Informed Practice (PIP) is advocated for physiotherapists managing individuals with chronic pain. Yet, there is a gap in research highlighting its real-world application. A study led by Denneny et al. explored the strategies used by physiotherapists in treating groups with chronic pain. They identified four primary objectives of physiotherapists: establishing a therapeutic relationship, diminishing perceived threats, reshaping beliefs and physical perceptions, and boosting self-confidence. The professionals also noted challenges, such as motivating patients for self-care, promoting activity, and emphasizing reinforcement over mere movement correction. The behaviours noticed in this study closely align with existing CBT techniques. Denneny's research enriches current guidelines by illustrating these techniques in real-world scenarios, advocating for enhanced training and mentorship to bolster the efficacy and confidence of physiotherapists in PIP (Denneny et al., 2020).

Chronic pain is not just prolonged acute pain. It often involves intricate interplays between physiological processes, psychological states, and socio-environmental factors. Emotions, thoughts, beliefs, and behaviours can amplify or alleviate a person's experience of pain, making the psychological domain an essential area of focus for physical therapists. Here, we will explore the importance of becoming a psychologically informed physical therapist and the steps to achieve this specialization.

BENEFITS OF A PSYCHOLOGICALLY INFORMED APPROACH

Becoming a psychologically informed physical therapist means going beyond the conventional boundaries of physical therapy and acknowledging the intricate interplay between the body and mind. Chronic pain, for instance, is not just a physical sensation but is often intertwined with emotions, past experiences, and personal beliefs. Recognizing this complexity is central to the psychologically informed approach.

1. Deepening Patient Understanding: A psychologically informed physical therapist does not see a patient's pain as just a symptom to be treated. Instead, they consider the whole individual – their fears, anxieties, past traumas, and current stressors. This allows for a deeper understanding of the root causes and influencing factors of a patient's pain experience.

2. Improved Patient-Provider Communication: Physical therapists can build a stronger rapport with their patients by being attuned to the psychological aspects of pain. This fosters trust, which is crucial for open communication. When patients feel understood and safe, they are more likely to share relevant information that can influence treatment outcomes.

3. Tailored Interventions: Physiologically informed care recognizes that two patients with the same physical ailment might require different therapeutic approaches based on their psychological profiles. One patient might benefit from mindfulness exercises to reduce anxiety-driven pain amplification, while another might need cognitive-behavioural strategies to tackle pain-related fears.

4. Enhanced Coping Strategies: Understanding the psychological facets of pain means therapists can equip patients with coping tools that address their physical and emotional needs. This might include relaxation techniques, stress-reduction strategies, or methods to reframe negative thoughts.

5. Promotion of Patient Autonomy: Empowering patients is a key aspect of the psychologically informed approach. By teaching them about the connection between mind and body and providing tools to manage their emotional responses to pain, therapists help patients regain a sense of control over their lives.

6. Professional Growth and Fulfillment: This holistic approach can lead to professional growth for the physical therapists themselves. As they integrate psychological principles into their practice, they broaden their skill set, making them more versatile and capable clinicians. Moreover, witnessing the profound impact of their work on patients' lives can bring immense professional satisfaction.

7. Reduced Risk of Chronicity: Addressing psychological factors early on, especially in cases of acute pain, can prevent the transition to chronic pain by breaking the cycle of pain and negative emotional responses.

8. Enhanced Multidisciplinary Collaboration: A psychologically informed approach often necessitates collaboration with other professionals, such as psychologists or counsellors. This multidisciplinary approach ensures comprehensive care for the patient.

9. Increased Patient Empowerment: By understanding and addressing the psychological factors influencing their condition, patients often feel more empowered and in control of their recovery journey.

10. Reduced Treatment Costs: Over time, addressing both the physical and psychological factors can lead to faster recovery rates and reduced need for extended therapy or interventions, potentially leading to cost savings.

In essence, a psychologically informed approach in physical therapy is a progressive step towards holistic patient care, recognizing the intricate interplay of mind and body in health and recovery. This holistic perspective ensures that therapy addresses the root causes of issues, leading to more lasting and comprehensive outcomes.

STEPS TO BECOME A PSYCHOLOGICALLY INFORMED PHYSICAL THERAPIST:

1. Education and Training:

 - Attend workshops, seminars, and courses that delve into pain science, cognitive-behavioural therapy, motivational interviewing, and other relevant psychological techniques.

 - Consider obtaining a postgraduate degree or certificate in health psychology, chronic pain management or a related field.

2. Clinical Experience:

During your clinical rotations or initial years of work, pay attention to the emotional and psychological aspects of your patients' experiences. This can help you recognize patterns and understand the psychological barriers to recovery.

3. Understand the Biopsychosocial Model:

This model emphasizes that health outcomes are influenced not just by biological factors but also by psychological and social aspects. Familiarize yourself with this approach, as it is foundational to becoming psychologically informed.

4. Cultivate Active Listening Skills:

 - Seek to understand, not just hear, your patients. This means paying attention to their verbal cues, non-verbal expressions, and the emotions behind their words.

5. Develop Patient-Centered Communication:

 - Use open-ended questions.

 - Validate their experiences.

 - Collaboratively set goals.

 - Provide clear and actionable feedback.

6. Incorporate Cognitive-Behavioral Strategies:

 - Educate patients about the pain experience and how thoughts, emotions, and behaviours can influence pain.

 - Help patients identify and challenge unhelpful beliefs or thoughts.

 - Incorporate relaxation and mindfulness techniques to reduce pain perception.

7. Integrate Motivational Interviewing Techniques:

 - Understand a patient's readiness for change.

 - Elicit and strengthen their intrinsic motivation.

 - Help them overcome ambivalence about change.

8. Stay Updated:

 - Pain science and psychological research continually evolve. Stay abreast of the latest findings and best practices through journals, seminars, and peer discussions.

9. Integrate Pain Science:

Understand the psychological aspects of pain. Pain isn't just a physical sensation; beliefs, emotions, and previous experiences also influence it. Familiarize yourself with current pain science to better assist patients who experience chronic pain.

10. Seek Supervision and Peer Feedback:

 - Engaging with mentors or peers can provide invaluable insights and ensure your approach remains patient-centred and evidence-based.

11. Collaborate with Mental Health Professionals:

If a patient presents with psychological challenges beyond your scope of practice, know when to refer them to a psychologist, counsellor, or psychiatrist. Establish a network of mental health professionals for collaboration and consultation.

12. Practice Self-Care:

Be aware of the emotional impact that engaging with patients in pain or distress can have on you. Delving into the emotional and psychological facets of pain can be emotionally demanding. Prioritize self-care and seek guidance or counselling to safeguard your mental well-being. Always remember to seek support when needed.

With this level of detailed immersion into each step, a physical therapist will develop a strong foundation in psychologically informed practices and foster deeper connections with patients. The ultimate aim is to craft a caring environment that is supportive, understanding, and evidence-based, catering to both the physical and psychological dimensions of pain and healing.

Becoming a psychologically informed physical therapist is about embracing a holistic approach to pain management. By understanding and integrating the psychological dimensions of pain, physical therapists can provide more effective, comprehensive care to their patients, fostering physical recovery and emotional and psychological well-being.

Key Message:

This chapter highlights the critical integration of psychological understanding into physical therapy to enhance therapeutic outcomes. By recognizing the interplay between physical ailments and psychological factors, therapists can provide more holistic and effective care. This synergy helps address the multidimensional nature of chronic pain, improve patient-provider communication, and promote patient autonomy. Through education, tailored interventions, and multidisciplinary collaboration, physical therapists can significantly improve their practice and patient well-being.

Reflection Exercise

Use the following questions as a guide for your reflection. Write your responses in the space provided or in a separate document. These questions can foster deeper understanding and collaboration between patients and health providers, ultimately leading to more effective chronic pain management.

FOR PATIENTS:

1. How do you think your mental and emotional state affects your physical pain or recovery process?

Response: _____

_____

_____

2. Do you feel comfortable discussing your mental health with your physical therapist? Why or why not?

Response: _____

_____

_____

3. How can your healthcare providers help you develop better coping mechanisms for your condition?

Response: _____

_____

_____

4. How much control do you feel you have over your recovery process? What can be done to increase this feeling?

Response: _____

_____

_____

For Health Providers:

5. What barriers do you face in integrating psychological aspects into your treatment plans?

Response: _____

_____

_____

6. How can understanding a patient's psychological state improve your communication and relationship with them?

Response: _____

_____

_____

7. What challenges do you face when incorporating psychological aspects into your practice?

Response: _____

_____

_____

8. How does a psychologically informed approach empower patients in their recovery journey?

Response: _____

_____

_____

True or False Questions

1. Integrating psychological understanding into physical therapy can enhance therapeutic outcomes.

2. Chronic pain is simply prolonged acute pain without any psychological components.

3. Physical therapists should only focus on the physical aspects of a patient's condition.

4. Psychological factors can influence the effectiveness of physical therapy treatments.

5. Building a strong patient-provider relationship is not crucial for effective physical therapy.

6. Addressing psychological aspects of pain can prevent the transition from acute to chronic pain.

7. Understanding a patient's psychological state can improve patient-provider communication.

8. Physical therapists can benefit from training in cognitive-behavioral therapy techniques

9. Only physical symptoms should be considered when treating chronic pain.

10. Teaching patients about the connection between mind and body can help them regain a sense of control over their recovery.

Answers

1. True

2. False

3. False

4. True

5. False

6. True

7. True

8. True

9. False

10. True

EMBRACING THE MIND IN THE JOURNEY OF PAIN: A PHYSICAL THERAPIST'S EVOLUTION

Amara had always known she wanted to be a physical therapist. Ever since her younger brother had injured his knee playing soccer, she had watched, fascinated, as he worked with a PT to regain his strength and mobility. When she finally opened her own clinic, she was elated. But as the years rolled on, she noticed a pattern: while many of her patients recovered, a significant number, especially those with chronic pain, seemed stuck, unable to make progress.

One such patient was Clara. An avid dancer, Clara had developed persistent lower back pain that stymied her every move. While her MRI showed some minor issues, the severity of her pain seemed out of proportion. They tried every treatment in the book - hot and cold packs, electric stimulation, manual therapy, and exercises, but nothing seemed to yield lasting relief. Clara was becoming increasingly frustrated and despondent.

One evening, after a particularly trying session with Clara, Amara sat down with a cup of tea, diving into a new book she had purchased on the intersections of psychology and physical health. The book delved into how our minds and emotions could amplify or alleviate our experiences of pain. A thought struck her - was Clara's pain, not just physical but also intertwined with her psychological state?

With this new insight, Amara began a journey to becoming a psychologically informed physical therapist. She attended workshops that explained the intricate interplay of mind and body in chronic pain. She learned about how fear, anxiety, past traumas, and even societal perceptions could feed into a person's pain experience. Techniques like cognitive-behavioural therapy, motivational interviewing, and mindfulness meditation became tools in her repertoire.

As she integrated these techniques, her sessions with Clara began to change. They started discussing not just her pain but her fears of never dancing again, the anxiety of a relapse, and the societal pressure she felt to always be at her best. Amara introduced Clara to deep breathing exercises and taught her to challenge her negative thoughts, slowly transforming them into positive affirmations.

Months later, the transformation was evident. Clara still had some pain, but it was manageable. More importantly, she had regained her joy of dancing. She understood her body better, listened to it more, and developed a healthier relationship with her pain.

Amara's clinic began to evolve. She now held workshops for patients, educating them about the mind-body connection. She collaborated with psychologists, inviting them to speak to her patients or refer those in need. Her success rates soared, and her patients, feeling heard and understood more holistically, became her biggest advocates.

Clara's journey had taught Amara a valuable lesson. Pain is not just a physical sensation; it's an experience deeply influenced by our minds. By embracing the psychological realm, Amara hadn't just become a better physical therapist; she had become a beacon of hope for those trapped in the maze of chronic pain.

Reflection Exercise:

1.   Why did Amara realize that traditional physical therapy methods were insufficient for treating chronic pain in some patients?

Response: _____

_____

_____

2.   What psychological techniques did Amara learn and integrate into her practice, and how did they impact her treatment of Clara?

Response: _____

_____

_____

3.   How did Amara's journey into becoming a psychologically informed physical therapist affect her professional growth and satisfaction?

Response: _____

_____

_____

4.   What lessons did Amara learn from Clara's journey that transformed her practice and approach to physical therapy?

Response: _____

_____

_____

Idea: Amara became a physical therapist inspired by her brother's recovery from an injury. Over time, she noticed traditional methods weren't enough for patients with chronic pain, like Clara. Realizing the importance of psychological factors, Amara learned cognitive-behavioural therapy, motivational interviewing, and mindfulness meditation. These techniques helped Clara manage her pain and regain her joy of dancing. Amara incorporated psychological assessments, patient workshops, and psychologist collaboration into her clinic, improving patient outcomes and professional satisfaction. Other therapists can apply these lessons by integrating psychological techniques, pursuing additional training, and collaborating with mental health professionals to provide holistic care.

EXPLORING THE LINK BETWEEN NUTRITION AND CHRONIC PAIN

"Let food be the medicine and medicine be the food."

- Hippocrates

Synopsis: *Chronic pain is a pervasive issue affecting millions of individuals worldwide, significantly impacting their quality of life and overall well-being. Traditional pain management often focuses on pharmacological and physical therapies, but emerging evidence highlights the critical role of nutrition in managing chronic pain. A balanced, nutrient-rich diet can influence inflammation, pain perception, and overall health, making it an essential component of a comprehensive pain management strategy.*

NUTRITION AND CHRONIC PAIN: A VITAL CONNECTION

Nutrition impacts chronic pain through several mechanisms, including inflammation modulation, hormone regulation, and maintaining a healthy gut microbiome. Chronic pain conditions such as arthritis, fibromyalgia, and neuropathy are often associated with chronic inflammation. Specific dietary components can either exacerbate or mitigate inflammatory processes in the body (Elma Ö, 2022).

Inflammation and Diet

Inflammation is a natural response to injury or infection, but chronic inflammation can contribute to ongoing pain. Diet plays a pivotal role in modulating inflammation. Anti-inflammatory foods like fruits, vegetables, nuts, seeds, and fatty fish can help reduce inflammation and pain. Conversely, diets high in processed foods, sugar, and trans fats can promote inflammation.

Key Anti-Inflammatory Nutrients:

Omega-3 Fatty Acids: Found in fatty fish like salmon, mackerel, and sardines, as well as flaxseeds and walnuts, omega-3 fatty acids are known for their anti-inflammatory properties. Studies have shown that omega-3 supplements can reduce pain and inflammation in conditions like rheumatoid arthritis (Calder, 2013)

Antioxidants: Vitamins A, C, and E, found in colourful fruits and vegetables, help reduce oxidative stress and inflammation. Research indicates that antioxidants can lower inflammatory markers and improve pain symptoms (Pérez-Belmonte, 2018)

Polyphenols: Present in foods such as berries, green tea, and dark chocolate, polyphenols have been shown to reduce inflammation. Evidence suggests that polyphenols can modulate inflammatory pathways and provide pain relief (Pandey, 2009).

Gut Health and Pain

The gut microbiome, the community of microorganisms in the digestive tract, plays a significant role in health and disease. An imbalance in the gut microbiome, known as dysbiosis, has been linked to increased inflammation and chronic pain. A fibre-rich diet, prebiotics, and probiotics can promote a healthy gut microbiome, potentially reducing pain and inflammation.

Foods for Gut Health:

Fiber-Rich Foods: Whole grains, fruits, vegetables, and legumes support a healthy gut microbiome. Dietary fibre has been shown to enhance gut health and reduce inflammatory responses (Makki, 2018).

Prebiotics: Foods like garlic, onions, and bananas feed beneficial gut bacteria. Prebiotics can improve gut barrier function and reduce systemic inflammation (Slavin, 2013).

Probiotics: Fermented foods such as yogurt, kefir, sauerkraut, and kimchi introduce beneficial bacteria into the gut. Probiotics have been found to alleviate symptoms in patients with irritable bowel syndrome and other inflammatory conditions (Hempel, 2012).

Blood Sugar Regulation and Pain

Stable blood sugar levels are crucial for managing chronic pain. Fluctuations in blood sugar can lead to spikes in inflammation and exacerbate pain symptoms. A diet low in refined sugars and rich in complex carbohydrates, proteins, and healthy fats can help maintain stable blood sugar levels.

Tips for Stable Blood Sugar:

Choose Complex Carbohydrates: Opt for whole grains, beans, and legumes over refined carbohydrates. Complex carbohydrates provide a slower release of glucose, preventing rapid spikes in blood sugar (Jenkins, 2002).

Balance Meals: Include protein and healthy fats with each meal to slow the absorption of sugars. This can help maintain energy levels and reduce inflammation (Nuttall, 1991).

Avoid Sugary Beverages: Reduce or eliminate the consumption of sugary drinks, which can cause rapid spikes in blood sugar. High sugar intake increases inflammation and pain (Hu, 2013).

Weight Management and Pain

Excess body weight can exacerbate chronic pain conditions, particularly those affecting the joints, such as osteoarthritis. Maintaining a healthy weight through balanced nutrition and regular physical activity can reduce the mechanical stress on the joints and lower overall inflammation.

Strategies for Weight Management:

Portion Control: Be mindful of portion sizes to avoid overeating. Eating smaller, more frequent meals can help manage hunger and prevent weight gain (Ello-Martin JA, 2005)

Nutrient-Dense Foods: Focus on foods high in nutrients but low in calories, such as vegetables, fruits, and lean proteins. Nutrient-dense diets can support weight loss and improve overall health (Rolls, 2009).

Regular Physical Activity: Combine a healthy diet with regular exercise to promote weight loss and improve overall health. Physical activity helps with weight management, reduces pain, and improves function in chronic pain patients (Hoffman et al., 2005).

Practical Dietary Recommendations for Pain Management

Implementing dietary changes can be challenging, but small adjustments can significantly impact pain management. Here are some practical tips:

Increase Fruit and Vegetable Intake: Aim for at least five servings of fruits and vegetables per day. These foods contain anti-inflammatory nutrients and antioxidants (He et al., 2007).

Choose Healthy Fats: Incorporate sources of healthy fats, such as avocados, nuts, and olive oil, while reducing trans fats and saturated fats. Healthy fats can help reduce inflammation and support overall health (Mozaffarian et al., 2006).

Stay Hydrated: Drink plenty of water to support overall health and help reduce inflammation. Proper hydration is essential for maintaining bodily functions and reducing pain (Popkin et al., 2010).

Limit Processed Foods: Minimize consumption of processed and packaged foods high in sugar, salt, and unhealthy fats. Processed foods are often linked to increased inflammation and pain (Monteiro et al., 2011).

Mindful Eating: Pay attention to hunger and fullness cues, and avoid eating in response to stress or emotions. Mindful eating can help regulate food intake and improve dietary choices (Kristeller & Wolever, 2011).

Key Message

Nutrition is a powerful lifestyle factor in the management of chronic pain. By adopting an anti-inflammatory diet, supporting gut health, regulating blood sugar, and maintaining a healthy weight, individuals can significantly improve their pain symptoms and overall quality of life. Integrating these nutritional strategies into a holistic pain management plan can lead to more effective and sustainable outcomes for chronic pain patients.

Reflection Exercise

Reflecting on this chapter highlights the important role of nutrition in managing chronic pain. By identifying areas for improvement and setting actionable goals, you can make meaningful dietary changes that may help reduce pain and improve your quality of life. Understanding the connection between nutrition and chronic pain is crucial for making informed dietary choices. Use the following questions and prompts to guide your reflection and write your responses in the provided space or a separate document.

For Patients:

1. How do you feel about making dietary changes to reduce inflammation and pain?

Response: _____

_____

_____

2. What changes can you make to include more nutrients in your meals?

Response: _____

_____

_____

3. How familiar were you with the concept of the gut microbiome before reading this chapter? What steps can you take to improve your gut health through diet?

Response: _____

_____

_____

4. What new strategies can you try to manage your weight and reduce pain?

Response: _____

_____

_____

5. Which dietary recommendations seem most feasible for you to implement immediately?

Response: _____

_____

_____

For Health Providers:

6. How do you currently educate patients about the relationship between diet and inflammation?

Response: _____

_____

_____

7. How do you support patients in managing their weight to reduce chronic pain?

Response: _____

_____

_____

FROM PAIN TO PEACE: EMMA'S NUTRITIONAL JOURNEY

Once upon a time, a woman named Emma lived in the peaceful village of Greensborough. Emma was well-loved by her neighbours for her cheerful disposition and willingness to help anyone in need. However, Emma harboured a secret that only her closest friends and family knew – she suffered from chronic pain. This relentless pain, stemming from fibromyalgia and arthritis, often left her feeling exhausted and defeated.

One day, while attending a community health seminar, Emma met Dr. Harper, a renowned nutritionist who was giving a talk on the connection between nutrition and chronic pain. Dr. Harper spoke passionately about how dietary choices could significantly impact inflammation and pain. Intrigued and hopeful, Emma decided to learn more.

Dr. Harper explained that chronic pain conditions like arthritis, fibromyalgia, and neuropathy are often linked to chronic inflammation in the body. She highlighted how certain foods could either exacerbate or reduce this inflammation. Emma learned that inflammation, while a natural response to injury or infection, could become problematic when it persisted over time, contributing to ongoing pain.

Dr. Harper emphasized the importance of anti-inflammatory foods. She spoke of the benefits of fruits, vegetables, nuts, seeds, and fatty fish, like salmon, which are rich in Omega-3 fatty acids. Emma was fascinated to learn that these nutrients could help reduce inflammation and pain. Conversely, diets high in processed foods, sugar, and trans fats could promote inflammation and worsen pain symptoms.

Feeling inspired, Emma decided to overhaul her diet. She started incorporating more Omega-3-rich foods like flaxseeds and walnuts into her meals. She added colourful fruits and vegetables to her plate to benefit from their antioxidants, like vitamins A, C, and E. She also began enjoying foods high in polyphenols, like berries, green tea, and dark chocolate.

Dr. Harper also introduced Emma to the concept of gut health. She explained that the gut microbiome, the community of microorganisms in the digestive tract, played a significant role in inflammation and pain. An imbalance in the gut microbiome, known as dysbiosis, could increase inflammation. Emma started eating more fibre-rich foods like whole grains, fruits, vegetables, and legumes to support a healthy gut. She also included prebiotics, such as garlic and onions, and probiotics from fermented foods like yogurt and kimchi.

As Emma continued her dietary journey, she learned about the importance of blood sugar regulation. Dr. Harper explained that stable blood sugar levels were crucial for managing chronic pain, as fluctuations could lead to spikes in inflammation. Emma began choosing complex carbohydrates, like beans and whole grains, over-refined sugars and balanced her meals with protein and healthy fats to slow sugar absorption.

Another critical aspect Dr. Harper discussed was weight management. Excess body weight could exacerbate chronic pain, especially in joints. Emma focused on portion control, opting for smaller, more frequent meals, and chose nutrient-dense foods high in vitamins but low in calories. She also started a gentle exercise routine to help with weight management and reduce pain.

Implementing these changes wasn't easy. Sometimes, Emma craved sugary snacks or felt too tired to prepare a healthy meal. But she persevered, motivated by the noticeable improvement in her pain levels and overall well-being. She stayed hydrated, minimized processed foods, and practiced mindful eating, paying attention to her body's hunger and fullness cues.

Over time, Emma's chronic pain became more manageable. She felt more energetic and positive. Her journey inspired many in Greensborough, and soon, the village saw a ripple effect of healthier dietary choices and improved quality of life among its residents.

Emma's story is a testament to the powerful link between nutrition and chronic pain. By making informed dietary choices and embracing small, consistent changes, she transformed her health and happiness, proving that hope and relief are possible despite chronic pain.

Reflection Exercise:

1. What did Emma learn about the relationship between inflammation and diet?

Response: _____

_____

_____

2. What is the gut microbiome, and how does it relate to chronic pain, according to Dr. Harper?

Response: _____

_____

_____

3. What changes did Emma make to her diet to help regulate her blood sugar levels?

Response: _____

_____

_____

4. What challenges did Emma face when trying to change her diet?

Response: _____

_____

_____

5. How did she stay motivated and overcome these challenges?

Response: _____

_____

_____

Simple Action Plan:

For Patients:

•   Set three specific, achievable dietary goals based on what you learned.

•   Create a method to track your dietary changes and their impact on your pain levels.

- Identify sources of support, such as health providers, nutritionists, or support groups.

For Health Providers:

- Develop educational materials or workshops to inform patients about the link between nutrition and chronic pain.

- Create personalized patient dietary plans based on their unique needs and health conditions.

- Establish follow-up routines to monitor patient progress and adjust dietary recommendations as needed.

Idea: Write a letter to yourself outlining your goals for improving your diet to manage chronic pain. Include strategies for overcoming potential challenges and how you will stay motivated and inspired by Emma's story.

NEUROPLASTICITY AND CHRONIC PAIN MANAGEMENT

"Chronic pain can change how the brain processes pain, but understanding neuroplasticity allows us to develop better pain management strategies."

-Lorimer Moseley

Synopsis: *Neuroplasticity, the brain's remarkable ability to reorganize itself by forming new neural connections throughout life, is crucial in understanding and managing chronic pain. This chapter explores how neuroplasticity can be harnessed to develop effective chronic pain management strategies. We will delve into the mechanisms of neuroplasticity, its relationship with chronic pain, and how various therapeutic approaches leverage this phenomenon to alleviate pain and improve patient outcomes.*

Understanding Neuroplasticity:

Neuroplasticity refers to the brain's capacity to change and adapt in response to experiences, learning, or injury. This adaptability is essential for learning new skills, recovering from brain injuries, and adjusting to new situations. Neuroplasticity involves several processes, including synaptic plasticity (the strengthening or weakening of synapses), neurogenesis (the creation of new neurons), and the reorganization of neural networks. (Siddall & Siddall, 2013)

In chronic pain, neuroplasticity can have both beneficial and detrimental effects. On the one hand, it enables the brain to adapt and potentially mitigate pain signals. On the other hand, maladaptive neuroplasticity can lead to the persistence and intensification of pain, even in the absence of ongoing injury (Petersen-Felix & Curatolo, 2002) .

Chronic pain often results from neuroplastic changes in the central nervous system. Conditions like neuropathic pain syndrome (Sator-Katzenschlager, 2014), complex regional pain syndrome (CRPS), fibromyalgia, and phantom limb pain are associated with alterations in brain structure and function. These changes can include increased excitability of pain pathways, reduced inhibition of pain signals, and the reorganization of cortical maps related to the affected body parts.

Research has shown that chronic pain can lead to a 'rewiring' of the brain, where areas associated with pain processing become more active and interconnected. This rewiring can make pain more persistent and less responsive to traditional pain relief methods. However, understanding these changes also opens up opportunities for targeted interventions that leverage neuroplasticity to reverse or mitigate these effects.

Therapeutic Approaches Leveraging Neuroplasticity:

1. Cognitive Behavioral Therapy (CBT):

 - Mechanism: CBT helps patients reframe negative thoughts and behaviours associated with chronic pain. By altering the psychological response to pain, CBT can induce positive neuroplastic changes, reducing the perception of pain and improving coping strategies.

 - Application: Patients engage in structured therapy sessions where they learn to identify and change dysfunctional thinking patterns, engage in relaxation techniques, and gradually increase their activity levels. (Lim JA, 2018)

2. Graded Motor Imagery (GMI):

 - Mechanism: GMI involves a series of progressive exercises designed to retrain the brain's perception and response to pain. It includes techniques such as laterality training, motor imagery, and mirror therapy, which help normalize brain activity and reduce pain sensitivity.

 - Application: Patients start by recognizing left and right body parts, moving on to imagining movements without actual movement, and finally, using mirror therapy to create the illusion of normal movement in a painful limb. (Moseley, 2004)

3. Mindfulness-Based Stress Reduction (MBSR):

 - Mechanism: MBSR combines mindfulness meditation and yoga to help patients become more aware of their thoughts, feelings, and body sensations in a non-judgmental way. This awareness can change brain structure and function, promoting relaxation and reducing pain perception.

- Application: Patients participate in an 8-week program with guided meditation practices, yoga sessions, and group discussions. Regular mindfulness practice helps rewire the brain to respond to pain more adaptively (Davidson, et al., 2003).

4. Physical Therapy and Exercise:

- Mechanism: Physical activity stimulates neurogenesis and synaptic plasticity, improving the brain's ability to manage pain. Exercise also releases endorphins and natural painkillers and helps maintain a healthy body weight, reducing strain on painful areas (Kempermann, et al., 2010).

- Application: Physical therapists design individualized exercise programs that include aerobic activities, strength training, and flexibility exercises. These programs aim to enhance physical function and reduce pain through regular, controlled movement.

5. Pain Neuroscience Education (PNE):

- Mechanism: PNE educates patients about the neurophysiological mechanisms of pain, helping them understand that pain is not always indicative of tissue damage. This knowledge can reduce fear and anxiety related to pain, leading to neuroplastic changes that decrease pain sensitivity.

- Application: Patients attend educational sessions to learn about pain science, how pain is processed in the brain, and strategies to manage it. This education empowers them to take an active role in their pain management (Louw, Diener, Butler, & Puentedura, 2011).

Key Message:

Neuroplasticity offers a robust framework for understanding and managing chronic pain. By leveraging the brain's ability to adapt and reorganize, various therapeutic approaches can provide significant relief and improve the quality of life for individuals with chronic pain. Cognitive Behavioral Therapy, Graded Motor Imagery, Mindfulness-Based Stress Reduction, Physical Therapy, and Pain Neuroscience Education are all effective strategies that utilize neuroplasticity to alter pain pathways and promote healing. As research continues to advance, these neuroplasticity-based interventions hold promise for developing even more effective chronic pain management techniques, ultimately transforming the lives of those affected by persistent pain.

Reflection Exercise:

True or False questions

1. Neuroplasticity refers to the brain's ability to adapt and reorganize itself in response to experiences, learning, or injury.

2. Maladaptive neuroplasticity can contribute to the persistence and intensification of chronic pain.

3. Cognitive Behavioral Therapy (CBT) does not utilize neuroplasticity principles in its approach to managing chronic pain.

4. Graded Motor Imagery (GMI) involves techniques such as laterality training, motor imagery, and mirror therapy to retrain the brain's perception of pain.

5. Mindfulness-Based Stress Reduction (MBSR) focuses on physical exercises to manage chronic pain.

6. Physical activity does not influence neuroplasticity and, therefore, has no significant impact on chronic pain management.

7. Pain Neuroscience Education (PNE) aims to reduce pain by educating patients about the neurophysiological mechanisms of pain.

8. The reorganization of cortical maps related to affected body parts is a feature of neuroplasticity observed in conditions like complex regional pain syndrome (CRPS).

9. Neuroplasticity can only have positive effects on chronic pain management.

10. Neurogenesis refers to creating new neurons, which is a part of the neuroplasticity process.

11. CBT can induce positive neuroplastic changes by helping patients reframe negative thoughts and behaviours related to chronic pain.

12. Regular mindfulness practice in MBSR helps rewire the brain to respond to pain more adaptively.

13. Physical therapists do not play a role in the neuroplastic changes that help manage chronic pain.

14. Pain Neuroscience Education (PNE) empowers patients by reducing fear and anxiety related to pain through education.

Answers:

1. True

2. True

3. False

4. True

5. False

6. False

7. True

8. True

9. False

10. True

11. True

12. True

13. False

14. True

UNLOCKING THE BRAIN'S POTENTIAL: THE IMPACT OF REGULAR EXERCISE ON NEUROPLASTICITY

Regular exercise is widely recognized for its myriad physical health benefits, including improved cardiovascular health, enhanced muscle strength, and weight management. However, its profound impact on the brain and nervous system, particularly in promoting neuroplasticity, is equally significant yet often overlooked. This chapter delves into how regular physical activity influences brain function, supports neuroplasticity, and enhances cognitive abilities and emotional well-being.

THE MECHANISMS OF EXERCISE-INDUCED NEUROPLASTICITY:

Neuroplasticity refers to the brain's capacity to change and adapt in response to new experiences, learning, and environmental factors. Exercise stimulates several biological processes that contribute to neuroplasticity:

1. Increased Blood Flow and Oxygenation:

Physical activity enhances cerebral blood flow, giving the brain more oxygen and essential nutrients. This increased perfusion supports the growth of new neurons and synapses and removes metabolic waste products that can impair neural function.

2. Release of Neurotrophic Factors:

Exercise triggers the release of brain-derived neurotrophic factor (BDNF), crucial for neurons' survival, growth, and maintenance. BDNF is vital for synaptic plasticity and essential for learning and memory. Other neurotrophic factors, such as nerve growth factor (NGF) and insulin-like growth factor 1 (IGF-1), are also upregulated during physical activity, promoting neuronal health and function.

3. Neurogenesis:

Regular aerobic exercise promotes neurogenesis, particularly in the hippocampus, a region critical for memory and learning. This process is essential for maintaining cognitive function and has been linked to improved performance in memory tasks and learning abilities.

4. Synaptic Plasticity:

Exercise enhances synaptic plasticity, the ability of synapses to strengthen or weaken over time in response to activity levels. Synaptic plasticity underpins learning and memory, enabling the brain to adapt to new information and experiences.

Cognitive Benefits of Regular Exercise:

1. Enhanced Memory and Learning:

Regular physical activity improves memory and learning capabilities by promoting hippocampal neurogenesis and increasing synaptic plasticity. Studies show that individuals who engage in regular aerobic exercise perform better on memory tasks and have greater hippocampal volume than sedentary individuals.

2. Improved Executive Function:

Exercise enhances executive functions, such as problem-solving, planning, and attention, due to increased BDNF levels and improved connectivity in the prefrontal cortex. This improvement is particularly beneficial for aging populations, as these cognitive abilities often decline with age.

3. Increased Creativity:

Physical activity can boost creativity and divergent thinking, likely due to enhanced brain connectivity and the release of neurotransmitters like dopamine and endorphins. Creative thinking is essential for problem-solving and innovation, making exercise a valuable tool for cognitive flexibility.

Emotional and Psychological Benefits:

1. Reduced Anxiety and Depression:

Regular exercise effectively reduces symptoms of anxiety and depression by increasing endorphin, serotonin, and other neurotransmitter levels that promote well-being. Exercise also reduces stress hormone levels like cortisol, improving mood and emotional regulation.

2. Enhanced Stress Resilience:

Regular physical activity builds resilience to stress by modulating the brain's stress response systems, strengthening the hypothalamic-pituitary-adrenal (HPA) axis, and enhancing prefrontal cortex function. Improved stress resilience improves emotional stability and coping mechanisms in challenging situations.

3.   Better Sleep Quality:

Exercise positively impacts sleep patterns, improving sleep quality and duration. Regular physical activity helps regulate the circadian rhythm and reduces insomnia symptoms. Better sleep, in turn, supports cognitive functions and emotional well-being, creating a beneficial cycle of health improvements.

Long-term Benefits and Neuroprotection:

1.   Reduced Risk of Neurodegenerative Diseases:

Regular exercise is associated with a lower risk of developing neurodegenerative diseases such as Alzheimer's and Parkinson's. The neuroprotective effects of exercise are linked to enhanced neuroplasticity, increased neurogenesis, and reduced inflammation in the brain. Physical activity helps maintain brain volume and function, delaying the onset and progression of age-related cognitive decline.

2.   Longevity of Cognitive Functions:

Lifelong engagement in regular physical activity supports sustained cognitive functions into older age, including preserving memory, attention, and executive functions. The long-term cognitive benefits of exercise highlight its importance as a preventive measure for cognitive decline.

Key Message:

The profound impact of regular exercise on the brain and nervous system underscores its importance beyond physical health. By promoting neuroplasticity, exercise enhances cognitive abilities, emotional well-being, and resilience to stress. The release of neurotrophic factors, increased neurogenesis, and improved synaptic plasticity are critical mechanisms through which exercise exerts its beneficial effects. Regular physical activity supports cognitive functions and emotional health and offers neuroprotective benefits, reducing the risk of neurodegenerative diseases and sustaining cognitive vitality throughout life. Integrating regular exercise into daily routines is a powerful strategy for enhancing overall brain health and well-being.

Reflection Exercise:

Reflect on the insights from the chapter to deepen your understanding of how regular exercise affects neuroplasticity and the brain. Use these questions to guide your reflection, and write your responses in the provided space or a separate document.

For Patients:

1.   Think about a time when exercising made you feel mentally sharper or emotionally better. Can you relate this to the increased blood flow and oxygenation to your brain discussed in the chapter?

Response: _____

_____

_____

2.   Reflect on how regular exercise might be promoting neurogenesis in your hippocampus. How does this make you feel about the importance of staying active?

Response: _____

_____

_____

3.   How has regular exercise impacted your memory and learning abilities? Provide specific examples of tasks or activities where you noticed improvement.

Response: _____

_____

_____

4.   How does exercise affect your mood and anxiety levels? Can you recall a time when physical activity helped alleviate feelings of depression or stress?

Response: _____

_____

_____

5.   How has regular exercise improved your sleep quality? Do you find it easier to fall asleep or feel more rested upon waking?

Response: _____

_____

_____

6.   Consider any barriers you face in maintaining a regular exercise routine. How can you overcome these obstacles to gain the neuroplasticity benefits discussed in the chapter?

Response: _____

_____

_____

7.   Reflect on how exercise supports cognitive functions as you age. How does this information influence your commitment to maintaining a regular exercise routine?

Response: _____

_____

_____

For Health Providers:

8.   How can you explain the concept of neuroplasticity to your patients to help them understand the importance of regular exercise for brain health?

Response: _____

_____

_____

9.   How might you design exercise programs that specifically aim to enhance neurogenesis in patients, particularly those with cognitive decline?

Response: _____

_____

_____

10. How can you assess and improve sleep quality in patients through exercise programs? What specific types of exercises have you found most effective?

Response: _____

_____

_____

11. How can you encourage lifelong engagement in physical activity to support sustained cognitive functions in your patients?

Response: _____

_____

_____

12. Consider the barriers patients might face in maintaining regular exercise. How do you help them overcome these obstacles and stay motivated?

Response: _____

_____

_____

BRAINS IN MOTION: RIYAN'S QUEST FOR NEUROPLASTICITY THROUGH EXERCISE

In a quiet suburban neighbourhood, nestled between the bustling city and the serene countryside, he has lived with a man named Riyan. Riyan was an ordinary man with an extraordinary curiosity about the workings of the human mind. He spent his days teaching biology at the local high school, but his nights were often filled with reading and research. His latest fascination was with the profound impact of regular exercise on the brain and nervous system.

Riyan's interest began one evening as he read an article about the surprising benefits of physical activity on neuroplasticity. Intrigued, he decided to delve deeper into this subject, discovering how exercise could influence brain function, support neuroplasticity, and enhance cognitive abilities and emotional well-being. This journey would change not only his life but also the lives of his students and community.

Riyan started his exploration with neuroplasticity, the brain's remarkable ability to adapt and change in response to new experiences. He learned that exercise was a powerful catalyst for this process. During his morning runs, Riyan pondered how physical activity increased blood flow and oxygenation to the brain, fueling its growth and maintenance. He imagined how every stride sent a rush of nutrients and oxygen to his brain, helping to grow new neurons and synapses while clearing away metabolic waste.

As Riyan dug deeper, he discovered the role of neurotrophic factors, particularly brain-derived neurotrophic factor (BDNF). Exercise triggered the release of BDNF, which was crucial for the survival and growth of neurons. This protein was the lifeline for synaptic plasticity, the foundation of learning and memory. Riyan was fascinated by how his daily physical activity was strengthening his muscles and his brain's capacity to learn and remember.

In his biology class, Riyan shared his newfound knowledge with his students. He explained how regular aerobic exercise promoted neurogenesis, particularly in the hippocampus, a region critical for memory and learning. He described the process of synaptic plasticity and how exercise could enhance the ability of synapses to strengthen or weaken over time, enabling the brain to adapt to new information and experiences.

One day, Riyan decided to introduce a new element to his teaching. He started a morning exercise program at the school, encouraging students and staff to participate. To his delight, the initiative was met with enthusiasm. Students who once struggled with memory tasks began to show remarkable improvement. Riyan attributed this to the increased hippocampal volume and enhanced synaptic plasticity fostered by their regular physical activity.

As the weeks passed, Riyan noticed more changes. Students were not only performing better academically but were also displaying improved executive functions. They were better at problem-solving, planning, and maintaining attention. Riyan knew this was due to the increased levels of BDNF and the enhanced connectivity in their prefrontal cortex, a region crucial for these cognitive abilities.

The most surprising change was in their creativity. Students who had never been interested in the arts began to excel in creative projects. Riyan explained to them how physical activity boosted creativity and divergent thinking, likely due to enhanced brain connectivity and the release of neurotransmitters like dopamine and endorphins.

The benefits of exercise extend beyond academics. Riyan noticed a significant reduction in anxiety and depression among his students. The endorphins and serotonin released during physical activity promoted well-being, while the reduced cortisol levels helped them manage stress better. The students were more resilient, emotionally stable, and better equipped to handle challenging situations.

Riyan experienced better sleep quality, supporting his cognitive functions and emotional well-being. He shared these benefits with his students, encouraging them to maintain a regular exercise routine to regulate their circadian rhythms and combat insomnia.

As years went by, Riyan observed the long-term benefits of exercise on his students. Those who continued to engage in physical activity had a lower risk of developing neurodegenerative diseases like Alzheimer's and Parkinson's. The neuroprotective effects of exercise were evident as these individuals maintained their brain volume and cognitive functions well into their older age.

Riyan's journey into the world of exercise-induced neuroplasticity had a ripple effect, transforming not just his life but also the lives of his students and the community. He had discovered a simple yet powerful tool for enhancing brain function, cognitive abilities, and emotional well-being. Through his efforts, Riyan unlocked the potential of regular exercise to build a healthier, happier, and more resilient community. And so, the once ordinary man had made an extraordinary impact, one step at a time.

Reflection Exercises:

Reflect on the story of Riyan, an ordinary man whose exploration of the benefits of regular exercise transformed his life and the lives of those around him. This reflective exercise will help you draw parallels between Riyan's journey and your own experiences while also considering how to apply these insights to enhance your well-being.

1. Reflect on a time when you were deeply curious about a subject or a concept. What sparked your interest? How did you begin your exploration?

Journal Prompt: "I remember when I first became interested in _____. It started when I read/experienced _____. My initial steps to learn more involved _____."

2. Think about a moment when you realized the broader implications of something you were exploring. How did this new understanding affect your perspective or actions?

Journal Prompt: "A pivotal moment in my learning journey was discovering that _____. This realization changed my perspective by _____ and influenced my actions by _____."

3. Consider your current relationship with physical activity. How often do you engage in exercise? How does it affect your mental and emotional well-being?

Journal Prompt: "My current exercise routine involves _____. I notice that after exercising, I feel _____ mentally and _____ emotionally. The biggest benefits I've experienced are _____."

4. Reflect on how you can integrate the concept of exercise-induced neuroplasticity into your life. What small changes can you make to your routine to enhance your brain function and emotional well-being?

Journal Prompt: "To incorporate exercise-induced neuroplasticity into my life, I plan to start by _____. This small change will help improve my brain function by _____ and my emotional well-being by _____."

5. Think about how you can share the benefits of regular exercise with others in your community. What steps can you take to encourage others to adopt a more active lifestyle?

Journal Prompt: "To share the benefits of exercise with my community, I can _____. Encouraging others to adopt a more active lifestyle will be beneficial because _____."

6. Imagine the long-term impact of incorporating regular physical activity into your life and encouraging others to do the same. How do you envision your future and the future of your community?

Journal Prompt: "In the long term, incorporating regular exercise into my life will help me _____. I envision that my community, if more active, will _____. The most significant change I hope to see is _____."

Idea: Reflect on the overall impact of Riyan's story and how his journey resonates with your own experiences and aspirations. Consider how you can use these reflections to change your life and community positively.

Journal Prompt: "Riyan's journey into exercise-induced neuroplasticity resonates with me because _____. His story inspires me to _____. Moving forward, I will _____ to build a healthier, happier, and more resilient life for myself and those around me."

Action Steps

1. Set a Goal: Identify a specific goal related to physical activity you want to achieve next month.

Example: "My goal for the next month is to engage in 10 minutes of aerobic exercise five days a week."

2. Create a Plan: Outline a plan to achieve this goal, including specific actions, schedules, and any support you might need.

Example: "To achieve my goal, I will schedule my morning exercise sessions before work. I will join a local running group for motivation and accountability."

3. Monitor Progress: Set up a system to monitor your progress and reflect on any changes you notice in your well-being.

Example: "I will keep a daily journal to track my exercise activities and reflect on how I feel mentally and emotionally. I will review my progress at the end of each week."

Remember, like Riyan, you have the power to make a significant impact on your life and the lives of others through the simple yet profound act of regular physical activity. Embrace the journey, and celebrate every step towards a healthier, more resilient you.

REDEFINING CHRONIC PAIN MANAGEMENT WITH PHYSICAL THERAPY INSIGHTS

"The human body is the best picture of the human soul."

-Ludwig Wittgenstein

Synopsis: Chronic pain, a multifaceted experience persisting beyond normal tissue healing time, affects countless individuals globally. Physical therapy plays a pivotal role in managing and often alleviating this pain. This chapter delves deep into the potential of physical therapy in chronic pain management and outlines key techniques for pain reduction.

The management of chronic widespread pain is a complex and challenging area in healthcare due to the lack of a universally accepted treatment protocol. Traditional rehabilitation programs, despite being standardized, often fail to deliver long-term functional benefits to patients with chronic pain. A significant number of patients undergoing these rehabilitation programs do not report lasting or clinically significant improvements. This has raised questions about the impact of various treatment aspects, such as the duration of the treatment and the specific components of the rehabilitation programs, on their effectiveness.

Typical treatment for chronic pain includes conventional physiotherapy interventions focusing on improving aerobic capacity, strength, and flexibility. However, interventions by physiotherapists and occupational therapists that aim to enhance patients' ability to perform activities of daily living (ADL) are less studied and documented, despite the fact that functional ability at the activity level is a key outcome measure for patients with chronic pain. This situation underscores a critical need for research into interventions that improve physical function and enhance the ability to perform ADLs. Additionally, the potential benefits of combining exercise-based approaches with other management strategies for chronic pain warrant further exploration (Amris K, 2019).

The IMPROvE study was designed to address these gaps. Its initial phase, a randomized waiting list-controlled trial, evaluated the impact of a standardized, two-week, group-based interdisciplinary rehabilitation programme on the ability of patients with long-standing CWP to perform ADLs. While this initial phase demonstrated a modest benefit in ADL performance six months after the intervention, there were no notable improvements in self-reported functional abilities or psychological outcomes.

Building on these findings, the second phase of the IMPROvE study aimed to assess whether a more comprehensive management strategy could yield better outcomes. In this phase, participants initially in the control group were offered the same two-week rehabilitation program, followed by an additional 16 weeks of occupational therapy or physiotherapy. The primary objective was to evaluate and compare the outcomes of this combined approach. The results showed that adding occupational therapy or physiotherapy to the initial two-week programme led to improvements in functional ability for most participants, assessed four weeks after the completion of the rehabilitation.

Furthermore, the second aim of this phase was to determine if the combined intervention (two-week programme followed by 16 weeks of additional therapy) was more effective than the two-week programme alone in achieving sustainable and clinically relevant improvements. This was evaluated 88 weeks from the baseline. The hypothesis was that a comprehensive, prolonged treatment approach would lead to greater improvements in ADL performance and self-reported mental well-being compared to a shorter rehabilitation program. This phase of the IMPROvE study was crucial in understanding the long-term effectiveness of different treatment modalities and durations for patients with chronic widespread pain (Amris K, 2019).

Physical therapy, as an essential component of comprehensive pain management, plays a crucial role in addressing chronic pain conditions. The primary goal of physical therapy in chronic pain management is to reduce pain, improve physical function, enhance quality of life, and empower patients with the skills and knowledge to manage their pain independently. It addresses underlying biomechanical deficiencies, improves joint alignment and muscle function, and educates patients about pain science.

Focusing on underlying biomechanical deficiencies is becoming a crucial part of managing pain, especially as chronic pain affects a significant portion of the population. This approach, rooted in the concept that pain, particularly chronic pain, often reflects deeper mechanical problems in the body, leads physical therapists and medical professionals to target these fundamental issues to provide more sustained and effective pain relief solutions.

Biomechanical deficiencies involve structural flaws or weaknesses in the body, including bones, joints, muscles, and connective tissue. These can arise from various causes, such as habitual poor posture, repetitive movements, injuries, congenital issues, or lifestyle choices. Common examples include conditions like scoliosis (a curvature of the spine), joint misalignments, muscle imbalances, and weaknesses in the shoulder girdle musculatures.

The first step in addressing these deficiencies involves a comprehensive physical therapy assessment and diagnosis. This typically includes physical examinations, medical history analysis, and differential diagnosis. The goal is to identify the location of pain and how biomechanical issues might be contributing to it.

Physical therapists play a key role in this process. They begin with a detailed evaluation of the patient's condition, including a comprehensive physical examination and possibly diagnostic tools like gait analysis or posture assessments. They identify specific biomechanical deficiencies contributing to the patient's pain or functional limitations.

Once these root causes are identified, physical therapists develop personalized treatment plans. This may include tailored exercises and stretches to strengthen weak muscles, improve flexibility, and correct imbalances; manual therapy techniques like massage and joint mobilization; postural training to reduce bodily strain; and possibly braces or orthotics to correct biomechanical irregularities. Treatment also involves pain management techniques such as heat or cold therapy and electrical stimulation.

A holistic approach is essential to treat the pain and understand the interaction and impact of various body parts on each other. For example, knee pain might be linked to hip muscle weakness, and treating the hip can alleviate knee issues. This comprehensive strategy extends to education and prevention, teaching patients about maintaining biomechanical health through regular exercise, proper lifting techniques, and weight management. Ongoing evaluation and adjustment of treatment plans ensure their effectiveness over time.

In conclusion, concentrating on biomechanical deficiencies represents a significant shift in pain management, emphasizing holistic, patient-centred care. By understanding and correcting these deficiencies, healthcare providers, particularly physical therapists, offer more effective, long-lasting relief from pain, improving their patients' overall quality of life. This approach highlights the interconnectedness of the body's structure and function, promoting a more comprehensive understanding of health and wellness.

Physical therapists also employ various pain alleviation techniques tailored to their patient's needs and conditions. Grounded in science and clinical experience, these methods aim to reduce pain, improve function, and promote healing.

One of the primary techniques is Manual Therapy, which includes hands-on approaches such as massage, joint mobilization, and manipulation. These methods are essential in decreasing pain, improving joint mobility, and facilitating better movement. Additionally, Therapeutic Exercises are developed to strengthen muscles, increase flexibility, and improve endurance. These exercises reduce pain by enhancing muscular support around painful areas and improving overall physical function.

Stretching is another key technique used by physical therapists. By employing various stretching methods, they work to increase flexibility and reduce muscle tension, which in turn helps alleviate pain. Heat and Cold Therapy are also utilized, where the application of heat increases blood flow and relaxes muscles for pain relief, and cold therapy or cryotherapy reduces inflammation and numbs areas of pain.

Electrical Stimulation, such as Transcutaneous Electrical Nerve Stimulation (TENS), uses low-voltage electric currents for pain relief. This technique is often used for chronic pain conditions or alleviating pain after injuries or surgeries. Using sound waves, therapeutic ultrasound delivers deep heat to soft tissues and joints, reducing pain, increasing circulation, and promoting tissue healing.

Aquatic Therapy, which includes performing exercises in a pool, offers unique benefits for pain relief. The buoyancy of water reduces stress on joints and muscles, while the resistance of water aids in strengthening muscles.

Postural Training and Ergonomic Education are integral to a physical therapist's approach. Educating patients about correct posture and ergonomic principles helps reduce pain caused by poor body mechanics during daily activities. Kinesiology Taping involves placing elastic therapeutic tape on the body to support muscles and joints, reduce pain, and enhance lymphatic drainage. Biofeedback is another technique that helps patients understand how their bodies respond to pain and teaches them to control physiological functions to reduce pain.

Neuromuscular re-education focuses on retraining muscles and the nervous system to function optimally, often employing techniques like functional electrical stimulation. Postural Training is also crucial, as poor posture can worsen chronic pain. Physical therapists guide patients in adopting postures that minimize strain and optimize biomechanics.

Mind-body approaches include Biofeedback, where patients receive real-time data on physiological functions, enabling them to control specific body parameters to reduce pain. Relaxation Techniques, such as deep breathing or progressive muscle relaxation, aid in decreasing muscle tension and pain. Guided imagery is another method involving concentrating on positive images to distract the mind from pain.

Cognitive Functional Therapy (CFT) is designed to manage disabling Low Back Pain (LBP) and other types of back pain and disorders. It analyzes behavioural psychology and movement patterns to identify factors associated with LBP. This approach allows therapists to explore various aspects of an individual's pain, considering their personal views. The goal is to help patients understand and manage their pain within the context of their activities and lifestyle.

CFT is particularly useful for patients with chronic pain and negative pain beliefs. It employs a clinical reasoning framework to identify modifiable factors based on personal characteristics and responses to pain. This helps patients become autonomous and self-manage their pain with a personalized treatment plan.

Progressive Muscle Relaxation (PMR) is a technique to reduce stress anxiety and manage chronic pain by systematically tensing and relaxing different muscle groups. It involves finding a comfortable position in a quiet place, focusing on slow and deep breathing, tensing each muscle group for 5-10 seconds from the feet up to the head, and then relaxing each muscle group for 15-20 seconds, noticing the contrast between tension and relaxation. This process continues until all major muscle groups are relaxed. PMR helps reduce physical tension, lower stress and anxiety levels, and enhance overall relaxation and mindfulness. PMR can be particularly beneficial for individuals with chronic pain as it promotes muscle relaxation, reduces pain perception, and improves overall pain management by interrupting the pain and muscle tension cycle. It can be practiced daily or as needed to manage stress, physical tension, and chronic pain.

Additionally, Pain Neuroscience Education helps patients understand the neurophysiological processes of pain, which can alter their perceptions and responses to pain, thereby reducing its impact. Research indicates that physical therapy can significantly lessen the frequency of migraines, though this conclusion is based on a limited number of studies. Pain neuroscience education (PNE) has emerged as a promising approach to treating migraine as a chronic pain condition. A 2023 study by Meise R. is the first to evaluate the effects of integrating PNE with physical therapy for migraine sufferers. The study discovered that combining PNE and physical therapy was more effective in reducing migraine frequency than physiotherapy alone. It underscored the importance of understanding pain neurophysiology, which might change pain perception and diminish fear associated with migraines. However, the study acknowledged limitations, such as the lack of a control group, and suggested further research for more definitive results.

Physical therapists also employ self-management strategies to empower patients in managing their pain, significantly enhancing their quality of life. This includes activity pacing, which involves breaking tasks into manageable steps with rest periods to prevent pain exacerbation, and home exercise programs, which are tailored routines for patients to perform at home, amplifying the benefits of therapy. Lifestyle modifications in areas like sleep, diet, and stress management are also pivotal. In their approach, physical therapists often collaborate with occupational therapists to optimize daily functions, psychologists to address emotional aspects of chronic pain, and pain specialists and physicians to ensure comprehensive care. Given the unique nature of each patient's experience with chronic pain, it's essential for therapists to continually assess and adjust treatment plans, remain cognizant of the psychological impacts of chronic pain, and ensure that treatments are patient-centred.

Physical therapy plays a pivotal role in chronic pain management, employing a range of techniques tailored to the specific needs and conditions of each patient. The primary objective of physical therapy in this context is not just alleviating pain but also addressing its root causes. This approach significantly improves patients' quality of life and their functional abilities. As a key element in managing chronic pain, physical therapy offers a holistic approach that integrates biomechanics, neuroscience, and personalized care. Physical therapists possess diverse techniques, positioning them uniquely to assist patients on their journey through pain. Their focus extends beyond mere pain relief to include patient empowerment. By adopting these strategies, physical therapy can markedly enhance the lives of many individuals dealing with chronic pain.

PHYSICAL THERAPY'S PIVOTAL ROLE IN CHRONIC PAIN JOURNEY

Anna's passage through the shadowy realms of chronic pain and her transformative healing journey underscores a narrative replete with complexity, addressing the multifaceted nature of pain encompassing physical, psychological, and social dimensions. Her world, once vibrant and untroubled, grew dim as she grappled with relentless lower back pain, a constant metronome dictating a life now circumscribed by limitations. Memories of uninhibited treks and lively salsa evenings grew faint, obscured by a growing accumulation of medical prescriptions and restless nights.

Anna's descent into chronic pain marked a stark transition from a life of joy and activity to one shadowed by suffering. Her condition, initially a mere physical anomaly, rapidly metastasized into an all-consuming force, undermining her identity and severing the ties to her once joyful existence. Each day reflected a life marred by pain, a relentless tempo of discomfort and restriction.

The diagnosis of chronic lumbar pain, a consequence of disc herniation, opened a Pandora's box of medical treatments, each with its promise of relief and inherent letdowns. Anna's journey through the healthcare system was a tapestry of hope and disillusionment, as each treatment offered fleeting solace, only to be succeeded by recurring pain and frustration. Medications provided temporary relief but clouded her mind, and the myriads of procedures and recommendations often fell short of her hopes for recovery.

Anna's venture into physical therapy represented a significant shift, not merely in treatment but in her understanding and approach to pain. Initially skeptical, her perspective began to change after meeting Samir, a physical therapist who introduced her to a holistic view of healing. This wasn't merely about physical maneuvers but encompassing an understanding of the body's narrative, transforming pain into a manageable element of her life.

Engagement with physical therapy became a journey of empowerment for Anna. Each session helped reclaim a piece of herself lost to pain, blending manual therapy, neuromuscular exercises, and cognitive education into a coherent strategy for managing her condition. These therapeutic encounters were not just about alleviating pain but about reconstructing her identity and autonomy, guiding her toward a hopeful and active life.

Anna's healing journey ignited a passion for advocacy, inspiring her to share her experiences and support others enduring chronic pain. Her narrative transcended personal recovery, advocating for a nuanced understanding of pain management and the profound benefits of physical therapy. Through her advocacy, Anna illuminated the path for others, promoting a message of hope and resilience.

Physical therapy provided Anna with lasting tools to manage her pain, allowing her to maintain an enriched quality of life. This journey is emblematic of the broader efficacy of physical therapy in chronic pain management, highlighting its role in symptom control and fostering a comprehensive, empowered approach to health.

In conclusion, Anna's story encapsulates the profound journey from suffering to healing, underscoring the essential role of physical therapy in chronic pain management. It's a narrative that goes beyond individual experience, advocating for a holistic, empathetic approach to healthcare that empowers individuals to navigate their pain and reclaim their lives.

Reflection Exercise:

Anna's story is a poignant narrative that highlights the transformative potential of physical therapy in managing chronic pain. Through her journey, we see the multifaceted nature of pain and the comprehensive approach required for effective treatment. Reflect on the following questions to deepen your understanding of this story and its implications for chronic pain management. Write your responses in the provided space or a separate document.

IDRIS HAFIZ

For Patients:

1. How did Anna's chronic pain affect her daily life and identity?

Response: _____

_____

_____

2. Reflect on a time when physical or emotional pain has impacted your ability to enjoy activities you once loved. How did it change your perspective on those activities?

Response: _____

_____

_____

3. Why do you think chronic pain often leads to feelings of frustration and disillusionment with the healthcare system?

Response: _____

_____

_____

4. Consider your own experiences or those of someone you know with medical treatments. What were the expectations versus the reality of those treatments?

Response: _____

_____

_____

5. Reflect on the role of a healthcare professional (like Samir) in changing a patient's outlook towards their treatment. Have you or someone you know experienced a similar transformation through the influence of a healthcare provider?

Response: _____

_____

_____

For Health Providers:

6. Think about the combination of manual therapy, neuromuscular exercises, and cognitive education in Anna's treatment. Why is it important to address both physical and psychological aspects of pain?

Response: _____

_____

_____

7. What lasting tools did physical therapy provide Anna to manage her pain and maintain an enriched quality of life?

Response: _____

_____

_____

8. Consider the long-term benefits of physical therapy beyond immediate pain relief. How can these benefits contribute to an overall better quality of life?

Response: _____

_____

_____

9. Reflect on the broader implications of Anna's story for the healthcare system. How can her journey inform improvements in chronic pain management practices?

Response: _____

_____

_____

10. Summarize your reflections on Anna's story. What key insights have you gained about chronic pain management and the role of physical therapy?

Response: _____

_____

_____

Idea: Anna's story highlights the transformative power of physical therapy in managing chronic pain. Overwhelmed by lower back pain and ineffective treatments, she found relief through a holistic approach introduced by her physical therapist, Samir. Anna regained her life and identity by combining manual therapy, exercises, and cognitive education. Her journey underscores the critical role of physical therapy in addressing both physical and psychological aspects of pain, advocating for a patient-centred, holistic approach.

PHYSICAL THERAPY METHODS AND APPROACHES FOR CHRONIC PAIN MANAGEMENT

Chronic pain management in physical therapy involves various methods and approaches designed to alleviate pain, improve function, and enhance the quality of life for patients. Among these methods, the McKenzie Method of Mechanical Diagnosis and Therapy (MDT), the Yass Method, Graded Motor Imagery (GMI), and Mulligan's Techniques are notable. This chapter explores these approaches and their roles in chronic pain management.

McKenzie Method of Mechanical Diagnosis and Therapy (MDT)

The McKenzie Method, developed by Robin McKenzie, is a comprehensive approach to spinal and extremity pain based on patient self-treatment and individualized assessment. It is particularly effective for conditions such as low back pain, sciatica, and cervical pain. The method involves the following key components:

1. Assessment and Classification:

 -Mechanical Diagnosis: This involves a detailed assessment to classify patients into subgroups based on their responses to specific movements and positions. The goal is to identify the movement patterns that exacerbate or alleviate symptoms.

 - Directional Preference: Patients are often classified according to the direction of movement that reduces or centralizes their pain (e.g., flexion, extension). (Hefford, 2008)

2. Therapeutic Interventions:

 - Self-Treatment: Empowering patients to manage their pain through specific exercises and movements that promote centralization or reduction of symptoms.

 - Progressive Exercise: Gradually increase the complexity and intensity of exercises to restore full function and prevent recurrence.

 - Postural Education: Teaching patients about proper posture and body mechanics to prevent future pain episodes.

3. Outcome Measurement:

 - Regular assessment of pain levels and functional ability to adjust the treatment plan as needed.

(Halliday MH, 2019) This systematic review investigated the efficacy of Mechanical Diagnosis and Therapy (MDT) for low back pain by comparing treatment effects between trials adhering to MDT principles and those that did not. The core principles of MDT include classification into diagnostic syndromes, intervention based on classification, and appropriate application of force. Analyzing studies up to June 2018, the review found that trials fully adhering to MDT principles showed significantly greater reductions in pain and disability—15.0 and 11.7 points, respectively, on a 100-point scale—compared to non-adherent trials. The findings suggest that consistent application of MDT principles leads to better outcomes in managing low back pain.

Mechanical Diagnosis and Therapy (MDT) is used to treat extremity problems, and accurate classification is important for effective treatment. (Takasaki H, 2017) This study looked at how reliably different examiners classify MDT cases using three methods: vignette reliability (using patient scenarios), concurrent reliability (multiple assessors observing the same assessment), and successive reliability (multiple assessors independently assessing the same patient at different times). Six high-quality studies were reviewed. The vignette method showed strong reliability (Kappa values ≥ 0.7), the concurrent method had mixed results (Kappa 0.45 to 1.0), and the successive method showed poor reliability (Kappa < 0.6).

This clinical practice guideline was developed by a panel of international experts who recommended managing knee OA regarding exercise. MDT was 'strongly recommended' as an intervention (Brosseau L, 2017)

Yass Method

The Yass Method, developed by Dr. Mitchell Yass, focuses on diagnosing and treating pain through a muscle-based approach. It emphasizes the role of muscular imbalances and weaknesses in chronic pain. The Yass Method involves the following principles:

1. Assessment and Diagnosis:

 - Muscle Testing: Manual muscle testing identifies specific weak or imbalanced muscles.

 - Symptom Interpretation: Understanding the nature of pain and correlating it with specific muscular dysfunctions rather than assuming structural damage (e.g., herniated discs).

2. Therapeutic Interventions:

- Targeted Strengthening: Developing a customized exercise programme to strengthen weak muscles and correct imbalances. This often involves resistance training and functional exercises.

- Pain Relief Through Muscle Balance: Alleviating pain by restoring proper muscle function and balance, which in turn reduces stress on joints and other structures.

3. Patient Education:

- Empowerment: Educating patients about the role of muscles in pain and how to manage their condition through exercise and lifestyle modifications.

Graded Motor Imagery Program

Graded Motor Imagery (GMI) is an innovative approach to managing chronic pain, particularly for conditions like complex regional pain syndrome (CRPS), phantom limb pain, and other persistent pain syndromes. GMI aims to retrain the brain and nervous system to alleviate pain and improve function. It involves a series of progressive stages that help patients regain normal movement and reduce pain perception. Here are the key components of the Graded Motor Imagery program:

1. Laterality Reconstruction:

- Objective: Improve the brain's ability to recognize left and right body parts. This stage is crucial because chronic pain can disrupt the brain's ability to correctly identify body parts, leading to increased pain and dysfunction.

- Method: Patients use images of hands, feet, or other body parts and practice identifying whether the images are of the left or right side. This can be done using flashcards, apps, or computer programs designed for this purpose.

2. Imagined Movements:

- Objective: Reintroduce the brain to the idea of movement without actually performing the movement, which helps to desensitize the nervous system.

- Method: Patients visualize themselves performing specific movements without physically moving. This mental rehearsal activates similar neural pathways as actual movement but without the risk of pain or injury.

3. Mirror Therapy:

- Objective: Use visual feedback to trick the brain into perceiving normal movement and reduce pain.

- Method: Patients perform movements with their unaffected limb while watching its reflection in a mirror, making it appear that the affected limb is moving normally. This visual illusion helps rewire the brain and decrease pain perception.

Mulligan's Techniques

Brian R. Mulligan qualified as a physiotherapist in 1954 and received his diploma in Manipulative Therapy in 1974. He has authored numerous articles published in the New Zealand Journal of Physiotherapy and two books: "Manual Therapy 'NAGS,' 'SNAGS,' 'MWMS,' etc." (2003) for physiotherapists, and "Self-Treatment for the Back, Neck and Limbs" for the public.

Mulligan's Techniques are manual therapy techniques that combine passive mobilization with active movement. They are designed to correct positional faults and improve joint function, providing immediate pain relief and improved range of motion (R.Mulligan, 2010).

During assessment and treatment, therapists look for the PILL response:

P: Pain-free

I: Instant result

LL: Long-lasting

If there is no PILL response, the technique should not be used.

The second principle is CROCKS:

C: Contra-indications (No PILL response is a contraindication)

R: Repetitions (Only three reps on the first day)

O: Overpressure

C: Communication

K: Knowledge (of treatment planes and pathologies)

S: Sustain the mobilization throughout the movement.

Mulligan's Techniques include:

1. Mobilization with Movement (MWM):

- Objective: Restore normal joint function by combining therapist-applied mobilization with patient-performed active movement.

- Method: The therapist applies a gentle, sustained mobilization to the affected joint while the patient performs a specific movement. This technique is often used for conditions like shoulder impingement, knee osteoarthritis, and ankle sprains.

2. Sustained Natural Apophyseal Glides (SNAGs):

- Objective: Improve spinal mobility and reduce pain through sustained gliding movements.

- Method: The therapist applies a glide to a spinal segment while the patient moves through a range of motion. This technique is particularly useful for neck and back pain.

3. NAGs (Natural Apophyseal Glides):

- Objective: Provide pain relief and improve spinal movement through oscillatory mobilizations.

- Method: The therapist performs gentle oscillatory movements to the spinal facet joints, which can be done in various positions depending on the patient's symptoms.

INTEGRATING VARIOUS TECHNIQUES AND APPROACHES IN CHRONIC PAIN MANAGEMENT

Integrating different physical therapy techniques can significantly enhance the effectiveness of chronic pain management. Let's explore how methods like McKenzie MDT, Mulligan's Techniques, the Yass Method, and Graded Motor Imagery (GMI) can be combined, sequenced, and used complementarily to provide comprehensive care.

1. Combination of Techniques: McKenzie MDT and Mulligan's Techniques

Imagine a patient named Sarah struggling with persistent lower back pain. We start with the McKenzie Method to perform a thorough mechanical assessment, identifying her directional preference—movements or positions that either alleviate or exacerbate her pain. Sarah finds relief in extension movements but not in flexion. This step is crucial as it personalizes her treatment plan, ensuring we focus on the most beneficial movements.

With this knowledge, we apply Mulligan's Techniques for immediate pain relief and improved joint function. Techniques like Mobilization with Movement (MWM) help correct positional faults and facilitate normal joint mechanics while Sarah performs active movements. For instance, if Sarah experiences pain while bending forward, a gentle glide the therapist applies during the movement can alleviate discomfort and restore normal function. This combination quickly alleviates her pain, allowing her to engage more effectively in subsequent exercises. This immediate relief is physical and psychological, boosting Sarah's confidence in her ability to move without pain.

Yass Method and GMI:

Next, consider John, who experiences chronic shoulder pain. We use the Yass Method to assess muscular imbalances and weaknesses, developing a targeted strengthening program. John begins specific resistance exercises to strengthen weak muscles and restore balance, which is crucial for alleviating his chronic pain caused by muscle dysfunction. This might involve exercises like resisted shoulder external rotations or scapular stabilization exercises tailored to his specific needs.

To complement this, we incorporate Graded Motor Imagery (GMI) to address central sensitization. We start with Laterality Reconstruction to improve John's brain recognition of body parts, followed by Imagined Movements to reintroduce pain-free movement patterns. Finally, Mirror Therapy creates visual feedback that promotes normal movement perception, further aiding John's recovery. This combination addresses both the physical and neurological aspects of his pain, providing a comprehensive approach to treatment.

2. Sequential Integration

Initial Phase:

Let's follow another patient, Emily, through her journey. Emily's pain sensitivity and fear of movement are significant barriers. We begin with GMI to tackle neural sensitization. Starting with Laterality Reconstruction and progressing to Imagined Movements and Mirror Therapy, Emily's pain perception is reduced, and her nervous system is prepared for physical activity. This phase is foundational, as it builds her confidence and reduces fear-avoidance behaviours, setting a positive tone for subsequent therapy.

Middle Phase:

In the middle phase, we implement Mulligan's Techniques to provide Emily with immediate pain relief and improve her joint mobility. Simultaneously, we use McKenzie's MDT to identify and reinforce her directional preference. This phase focuses on reducing pain through manual therapy and promoting movements that align with Emily's directional preference. For example, if Emily has neck pain that improves with retraction movements, we use Mulligan's sustained glides during these retraction movements to enhance pain relief and mobility.

Final Phase:

As we conclude Emily's treatment, we focus on the Yass Method, aiming for long-term muscular strengthening and balance. We ensure that Emily achieves sustained functional improvement by addressing any remaining muscular imbalances, reducing the likelihood of pain recurrence. This phase might include progressive resistance training and functional exercises tailored to her daily activities, ensuring she can maintain the improvements gained during therapy.

3. Complementary Use

Manual Therapy and Therapeutic Exercise:

Consider Mark, who combines manual therapy techniques like Mulligan's MWM with the McKenzie MDT and Yass Method therapeutic exercises. After using MWM to alleviate immediate pain and improve joint function, Mark follows up with McKenzie exercises that align with his directional preference to maintain joint mobility. Incorporating Yass Method exercises strengthens the surrounding musculature, providing a comprehensive approach to pain management. This integrated approach ensures that Mark experiences immediate relief and builds long-term resilience against future pain episodes.

Patient Education and Cognitive Approaches:

Finally, we have Lisa, who benefits from education in pain management. We explain the role of the brain in pain perception (GMI), the importance of muscle balance (Yass Method), and the benefits of self-treatment strategies (McKenzie MDT). This knowledge empowers Lisa to understand her condition better and actively participate in her rehabilitation. Integrating cognitive-behavioural approaches addresses the psychological aspects of chronic pain, enhancing the effectiveness of physical therapy interventions; by teaching Lisa coping strategies, stress management, and how thoughts and emotions impact pain, we provide her with tools to manage her pain more effectively, both during and after her rehabilitation.

The McKenzie Method provides a systematic approach to identifying and addressing directional preference, which helps centralize and reduce pain through specific movements and exercises. Its emphasis on self-treatment empowers patients, giving them tools to manage their pain independently. This self-sufficiency is crucial for long-term management, as patients learn to control their symptoms without constant therapist intervention.

The Yass Method focuses on identifying and correcting muscular imbalances, a common but often overlooked source of chronic pain. By strengthening weak muscles and restoring balance, this method addresses the root cause of pain rather than just the symptoms, promoting long-term recovery and prevention of recurrence. This holistic approach ensures that patients are treated for their pain and are equipped to prevent future episodes.

Graded Motor Imagery offers a novel approach to managing pain through neural desensitization and re-education of movement. By starting with cognitive techniques like laterality recognition and progressing through imagined movements to mirror therapy, GMI helps patients reduce pain perception and fear of movement, facilitating a smoother transition to physical rehabilitation. This cognitive-physical approach bridges the gap between mind and body, addressing pain comprehensively.

Mulligan's Techniques provide immediate pain relief and improved joint function through manual therapy combining passive and active mobilization. This immediate feedback and relief can enhance patient compliance and readiness for other therapeutic exercises. The rapid pain relief achieved through these techniques boosts patient morale and engagement, which are critical factors in the success of long-term therapy programs.

The integration of these methods leverages their strengths, creating a comprehensive and holistic approach to chronic pain management. Physical therapists can create a structured yet flexible treatment plan by starting with neural desensitization through GMI, progressing to manual therapy and mechanical diagnosis with Mulligan's Techniques and the McKenzie Method, and finally addressing muscle imbalances with the Yass Method. This integrative approach ensures that all patient pain aspects are addressed, leading to more effective and lasting relief.

While each of these methods is well-supported by research and literature in the field of physical therapy and rehabilitation, the specific strategies for their integration presented here are based on my own clinical experiences with chronic pain patients. Over years of practice, I have found that strategically combining these approaches addresses the multifactorial nature of chronic pain and enhances patient engagement and outcomes. This personalized and adaptive approach ensures that patients receive the most effective and comprehensive care possible, significantly improving their pain levels, function, and overall quality of life. We can achieve the best possible outcomes in chronic pain management by continuously adapting and refining these techniques based on individual patient responses.

Key Message

Chronic pain management in physical therapy is a multifaceted process that requires the use of various methods and approaches tailored to the individual needs of patients. The McKenzie Method, Yass Method, Graded Motor Imagery (GMI), and Mulligan's Techniques each offer unique strategies that, when integrated, can effectively address chronic pain.

Reflection Exercise

Reflecting on this chapter highlights that chronic pain management in physical therapy is a multifaceted process requiring various methods and approaches tailored to patients' individual needs. Use the following questions and prompts to guide your reflection, and write your responses in the provided space or a separate document.

For Patients:

1.   Reflect on the various pain management strategies you have tried in the past. Which ones have provided the most relief? Why do you think these methods were effective?

Response: _____

_____

_____

2.   Think about a typical day in your life. How does your current physical therapy intervention help you perform daily tasks? Are there any exercises that seem more beneficial than others?

Response: _____

_____

_____

3.   Reflect on any changes in your ability to perform activities of daily living (ADLs) since starting physical therapy. Have you noticed any improvements? If so, describe them.?

Response: _____

_____

_____

4.   Reflect on your understanding of your own biomechanical deficiencies. Have you discussed these with your physical therapist? What steps have you taken to address these issues?

Response: _____

_____

_____

5.   Reflect on any lifestyle changes you've made (e.g., diet, sleep, stress management) as part of your pain management plan. How have these changes affected your overall well-being?

Response: _____

_____

_____

For Health Providers:

6.   Reflect on the effectiveness of the traditional rehabilitation programs you currently use for chronic pain patients. Are there specific components that consistently show better outcomes?

Response: _____

_____

_____

7. Consider the duration and structure of your treatment protocols. How might extending the duration or modifying the components improve patient outcomes?

Response: _____

_____

_____

8. Think about the balance between improving physical function and enhancing ADLs. How can you ensure that your interventions are addressing both aspects effectively?

Response: _____

_____

_____

9. Consider the potential benefits of combining different therapeutic approaches in your practice. How can you implement a more comprehensive management strategy?

Response: _____

_____

_____

10. Think about the long-term outcomes of your patients. How can you adjust your treatment approaches to ensure sustainable and clinically relevant improvements in their pain management?

Response: _____

_____

_____

IDRIS HAFIZ

OPTIMIZING MUSCULOSKELETAL HEALTH: A PHYSIOTHERAPY APPROACH TO POSTURE AND PAIN BEHAVIORS

Posture, defined as the alignment and positioning of the body concerning gravity, plays a crucial role in overall musculoskeletal health. Pain behaviours, on the other hand, are observable actions or reactions that indicate the presence of pain. From a physiotherapy perspective, understanding the intricate relationship between posture and pain behaviours is essential for effective diagnosis, treatment, and prevention of musculoskeletal disorders. This chapter delves into the physiological and psychological aspects of posture and pain behaviours, emphasizing the vital role of physiotherapy in managing these components to enhance overall well-being.

The role of postural loads as a risk factor for back pain and musculoskeletal symptoms remains uncertain. In his classification of mechanical syndromes, McKenzie introduced the concept of postural syndrome, where individuals experience symptoms only from sustained loading that are relieved by changing positions without affecting movement or function. Due to the low level of disability associated with postural syndrome, it is suggested that few individuals seek healthcare for this issue (May, Nanche, & Pingle, 2011).

The Importance of Posture

Proper posture is fundamental for maintaining musculoskeletal health. It minimizes the strain on muscles, ligaments, and joints, thereby reducing the risk of injury and chronic pain. Good posture aligns the body so that the least strain is placed on supporting muscles and ligaments during movement or weight-bearing activities. The literature suggests that forward head posture (FHP) leads to increased thoracic kyphosis and changes in scapular positioning (downward rotation, anterior tilt, and protraction), causing greater compression in the subacromial space. These changes are often linked with muscle imbalances, and conservative rehabilitation typically addresses both posture and muscle balance. However, evidence supporting the role of posture and muscle imbalance in causing subacromial impingement syndrome (SIS) is limited. This study examined whether FHP is associated with increased thoracic kyphosis, altered scapular position, and reduced glenohumeral elevation in 60 asymptomatic individuals and 60 SIS patients. The results indicated that upper body posture does not always follow the patterns described in the literature (Lewis, Green, & Wright, 2005).

Types of Posture

1. Static Posture: This refers to how we hold ourselves when not moving, such as sitting, standing, or lying down. Activities requiring prolonged periods in one position, such as working at a desk or sleeping, are crucial.

2. Dynamic Posture: This involves the body's alignment during movement, such as walking, running, or lifting. Dynamic posture is essential for maintaining balance and preventing injuries during physical activities.

Posture and Its Impact on Pain

Improper posture can lead to a variety of musculoskeletal issues. Common problems associated with poor posture include back, neck, and shoulder pain. These issues often arise from prolonged static postures or repetitive movements that strain-specific muscle groups.

Mechanisms of Pain

1. Muscle Imbalance: Poor posture can cause certain muscles to become overactive while others become underactive, leading to imbalances that result in pain. For instance, prolonged sitting with a forward head posture can cause the neck extensors to become overactive while the deep neck flexors become underactive, resulting in neck pain.

2. Joint Misalignment: Incorrect posture can lead to improper joint alignment, causing increased wear and tear on the joints and leading to pain. An example is the increased lumbar lordosis often seen in individuals with anterior pelvic tilt, which can cause lower back pain.

3. Nerve Compression: Slouching or incorrect positioning can compress nerves, leading to pain and discomfort. For example, a slouched posture can compress the sciatic nerve, leading to sciatica.

Assessing Posture

Physiotherapists use various tools and techniques to assess posture. These include visual observation, palpation, and technology such as digital posture analysis tools. An accurate assessment helps in identifying postural deviations and their potential link to pain behaviours.

Assessment Techniques

1. Visual Observation: The physiotherapist observes the patient's posture from different angles (anterior, posterior, and lateral views) to identify any visible misalignments.

2. Palpation: The physiotherapist uses their hands to feel for any abnormalities in the alignment of the spine, pelvis, and other joints.

3. Digital Posture Analysis: Advanced tools, such as digital posture analysis software, can provide detailed information about the patient's posture, including angles of deviation and areas of strain.

Pain Behaviors and Their Significance

Pain behaviours are actions or reactions that indicate the presence of pain. These behaviours can be both conscious and unconscious and include vocal expressions (groaning, crying), facial expressions (grimacing), and protective movements (limping, bracing).

Types of Pain Behaviors

1. Verbal Expressions: Patients may describe their pain verbally, providing insights into its nature and intensity. For instance, patients might describe their pain as sharp, dull, or throbbing.

2. Non-Verbal Expressions: Facial expressions, body movements, and changes in posture can indicate pain. A patient might grimace or wince when moving a particular body part.

3. Protective Behaviors: These include avoiding or minimizing pain, such as favouring one side of the body or using assistive devices. For example, a patient with knee pain might limp to avoid putting weight on the affected leg.

The Role of Physiotherapy in Managing Posture and Pain Behaviors

Physiotherapy plays a critical role in addressing posture-related pain and modifying pain behaviours. The approach involves a combination of education, manual therapy, exercise prescription, and behavioural strategies.

Educational Interventions

Educating patients about the importance of good posture and the mechanisms of pain can empower them to take an active role in their recovery. This includes teaching proper ergonomic practices and body mechanics.

1. Ergonomic Education: Patients learn how to set up their workstations to promote good posture, including the correct height of chairs and computer screens.

2. Body Mechanics Training: Patients are taught how to perform daily activities, such as lifting and carrying objects, in ways that minimize strain on the body.

Manual Therapy

Manual therapy techniques, such as joint mobilizations, soft tissue massage, and myofascial release, can help correct postural imbalances and alleviate pain.

1. Joint Mobilizations: Gentle movements applied to joints can improve their range of motion and alignment.

2. Soft Tissue Massage: Massage techniques can reduce muscle tension and improve circulation.

3. Myofascial Release: This technique targets the fascia, the connective tissue surrounding muscles, to reduce pain and improve mobility.

Exercise Prescription

Tailored exercise programs are designed to strengthen weak muscles, stretch tight muscles, and improve overall flexibility and alignment. These programs may include core strengthening, stretching exercises, and proprioceptive training.

1. Core Strengthening: Exercises such as planks and bridges can strengthen the core muscles, providing better support for the spine.

2. Stretching Exercises: Stretching tight muscles, such as the hamstrings and hip flexors, can improve posture and reduce pain.

3. Proprioceptive Training: Exercises that improve balance and coordination can enhance dynamic posture and prevent injuries.

Behavioural Strategies

Cognitive-behavioural therapy (CBT) and other behavioural strategies can help patients modify pain behaviours and cope more effectively with chronic pain. This includes techniques for relaxation, stress management, and pain desensitization.

1. Relaxation Techniques: Practices such as deep breathing and progressive muscle relaxation can reduce muscle tension and pain.

2. Stress Management: Strategies such as mindfulness and meditation can help patients manage stress, which can exacerbate pain.

3. Pain Desensitization: Gradual exposure to movements and activities that cause pain can help desensitize the nervous system and reduce pain over time.

Key Message:

Understanding the relationship between posture and pain behaviours is essential for effective physiotherapy intervention. By addressing postural issues and modifying pain behaviours, physiotherapists can significantly reduce pain and improve the quality of life for their patients. This holistic approach targets the physical aspects of pain and empowers patients through education and behavioural modification, leading to sustainable long-term outcomes.

A Journey to Musculoskeletal Health: Mia's Story

Mia had always considered herself a healthy individual. Active in her youth, she played sports and maintained a generally healthy lifestyle. However, the demands of her office job had gradually taken a toll on her body. She often found herself slouched over her desk for hours, her neck craning forward to focus on her computer screen. Over time, she began experiencing persistent neck and back pain, which only worsened despite her efforts to adjust her posture. Unbeknownst to her, she was suffering from a condition known as forward head posture (FHP), which had significant implications for her musculoskeletal health.

Mia's pain behaviours were becoming more noticeable. She frequently rubbed her neck, grimaced in pain when she moved her shoulders, and sometimes avoided certain movements altogether. Her discomfort led her to seek the help of a physiotherapist, hoping to find relief.

Her physiotherapist, Deniel, began with a thorough assessment of her posture and pain behaviours. He explained that posture plays a crucial role in musculoskeletal health. Proper posture minimizes strain on muscles, ligaments, and joints, reducing the risk of injury and chronic pain. Poor posture, however, could lead to various issues, including back, neck, and shoulder pain.

Deniel used a combination of visual observation, palpation, and digital posture analysis to assess Mia's posture. He noted her increased thoracic kyphosis, the forward head position, and the protracted scapulae—all classic signs of FHP. These postural deviations had led to muscle imbalances and nerve compression, contributing to her pain.

Deniel explained that FHP often results in increased thoracic kyphosis and changes in scapular positioning, causing greater compression in the subacromial space. These changes are linked with muscle imbalances, where specific muscles become overactive while others weaken. For Mia, this meant her neck extensors were overworked, while her deep neck flexors were underactive, leading to neck pain.

Together, they formulated a comprehensive treatment plan. Deniel emphasized that the key to Mia's recovery was addressing her posture and muscle imbalances. The plan involved a combination of education, manual therapy, exercise, and behavioural strategies.

1. Ergonomic Education: Mia learned how to set up her workstation to promote good posture. She adjusted her chair height, positioned her computer screen at eye level, and used a lumbar support cushion.

2. Body Mechanics Training: Deniel taught Mia how to perform daily activities in ways that minimized strain on her body. She learned proper lifting techniques and how to maintain good posture during various activities.

3. Manual Therapy: Deniel used joint mobilizations and soft tissue massage to alleviate muscle tension and improve alignment. Myofascial release techniques targeted the fascia, reducing pain and enhancing mobility.

4. Exercise Prescription: Mia followed a tailored exercise programme designed to strengthen her weak muscles, stretch tight ones, and improve overall flexibility and alignment. She performed core strengthening exercises like planks and bridges and stretched her hamstrings and hip flexors to improve her posture.

5. Behavioural Strategies: To help Mia cope with pain, Deniel introduced her to cognitive-behavioural therapy (CBT) techniques. She practiced relaxation methods such as deep breathing and progressive muscle relaxation to reduce stress and muscle tension. Gradual exposure to movements that caused pain helped desensitize her nervous system over time.

As Mia diligently followed her treatment plan, she noticed significant improvements. Her pain behaviours diminished as her posture improved and her muscles became more balanced. She no longer grimaced with every movement, and the chronic ache in her neck and back subsided.

One day, Deniel presented Mia with two case studies to illustrate her progress. The first case involved a 45-year-old office worker with chronic lower back pain, much like Mia's situation. The patient had a pronounced anterior pelvic tilt and rounded shoulders, and their treatment included ergonomic education, core strengthening exercises, and manual therapy. The second case was a 30-year-old with frequent headaches and neck pain who benefitted from postural correction exercises, neck muscle stretches, and relaxation techniques.

Mia's journey highlighted the importance of understanding the relationship between posture and pain behaviours for effective physiotherapy intervention. By addressing her postural issues and modifying her pain behaviours, Mia significantly reduced her pain and improved her quality of life. She felt empowered by the education and behavioural modifications she had learned, leading to sustainable long-term outcomes.

As research in physiotherapy continues to evolve, integrating advanced technologies, such as virtual reality for posture correction and personalized treatment plans based on genetic and biomechanical assessments, promises even greater advancements. The collaboration between physiotherapists, healthcare providers, and researchers is crucial in advancing the understanding and management of posture and pain behaviours, ultimately enhancing patient care and outcomes.

Mia's story is a testament to the power of physiotherapy in transforming lives through optimizing musculoskeletal health.

Reflection Exercise:

Reflective exercises for patients and health providers are designed to promote a deeper understanding of posture and pain behaviours, encouraging proactive steps toward better musculoskeletal health. Patients and health providers can work together to achieve optimal outcomes by reflecting on personal habits and professional practices.

For patients:

1. Describe your typical posture throughout the day (e.g., sitting at a desk, standing, walking).

Response: _____

_____

_____

2. Have you noticed any patterns of discomfort or pain associated with your posture? If so, where and when do you feel this pain?

Response: _____

_____

_____

3. What actions or reactions do you exhibit when you experience pain (e.g., rubbing, grimacing, avoiding certain movements)?

Response: _____

_____

_____

4. How do these pain behaviours affect your daily life and activities?

Response: _____

_____

_____

5. How can you incorporate regular breaks and movements into your routine to prevent prolonged static postures?

Response: _____

_____

_____

6. Reflect on any exercises or stretches you currently do. Are they helping to improve your posture and reduce pain?

Response: _____

_____

_____

7. What new exercises or stretches can you incorporate to strengthen weak muscles and stretch tight ones?

Response: _____

_____

_____

8. How does stress impact your posture and pain levels?

Response: _____

_____

_____

9. What relaxation techniques (e.g., deep breathing, progressive muscle relaxation) can you practice to manage stress and reduce pain?

Response: _____

_____

_____

10. Based on Mia's story and reflections, set three achievable goals to improve your posture and musculoskeletal health.

Response: _____

_____

_____

11. How will you track your progress and stay motivated to achieve these goals?

Response: _____

_____

_____

For Health Providers:

12. How do you currently assess posture and pain behaviours in your patients?

Response: _____

_____

_____

13. Reflect on a recent patient case where posture and pain behaviours were significant factors. What treatment strategies did you use?

Response: _____

_____

_____

14. How do you educate your patients about the importance of posture and the mechanisms of pain?

Response: _____

_____

_____

15. What key factors do you consider when tailoring exercise programs to individual patients?

Response: _____

_____

_____

Idea:

As research in the field of physiotherapy continues to evolve, future directions may include the integration of advanced technologies such as virtual reality for posture correction and pain management, as well as the development of personalized treatment plans based on genetic and biomechanical assessments. The ongoing collaboration between physiotherapists, healthcare providers, and researchers will advance our understanding and management of posture and pain behaviours, ultimately enhancing patient care and outcomes.

There is some disagreement on the role posture plays in pain. To gain a deeper understanding and explore the different perspectives, check out the last section of the book, Pain Solutions: A Strategic Guide to Managing and Reducing Pain.

PROGRESSIVE MUSCLE RELAXATION IN PHYSIOTHERAPY FOR PAIN MANAGEMENT

Progressive Muscle Relaxation (PMR) is a relaxation technique that involves the systematic tensing and relaxing of various muscle groups in the body. Originally developed by Dr. Edmund Jacobson in 1934, PMR aims to reduce muscle tension, decrease stress, and alleviate pain (McCallie, Blum, & Hood, 2006). From a physiotherapy perspective, PMR is a valuable tool in pain management, offering a non-invasive and effective approach to reducing discomfort and improving overall well-being. This section explores the principles, applications, and benefits of PMR in physiotherapy for pain management (Dolbier & Rush, 2012).

Principles of Progressive Muscle Relaxation

PMR is based on the concept that muscle tension is often a response to stress and anxiety, and by consciously tensing and then relaxing muscles, individuals can achieve a deeper state of relaxation. The technique involves focusing on specific muscle groups, contracting them for a few seconds, and then releasing the tension while concentrating on the sensation of relaxation.

Steps in PMR

1. Preparation: The individual should find a quiet, comfortable place to sit or lie down. It's important to wear loose, comfortable clothing and remove any distractions.

2. Breathing: Deep, slow breathing is encouraged throughout the session to enhance relaxation. The individual should take slow, deep breaths through the nose and exhale slowly through the mouth.

3. Tensing and Relaxing: Starting from the toes and working up to the head, each muscle group is tensed for about 5-10 seconds and then relaxed for 15-20 seconds. The process includes:

- Feet and toes

- Calves

- Thighs

- Buttocks

- Abdomen

- Chest

- Hands and forearms

- Upper arms

- Shoulders

- Neck

- Face (including jaw, eyes, and forehead)

4. Focus on Sensation: After tensing and relaxing each muscle group, the individual should focus on the contrast between tension and relaxation and the following sensation of calm.

Applications of PMR in Physiotherapy

PMR can be integrated into physiotherapy sessions to help manage pain, particularly in patients with chronic pain conditions. It is part of a holistic approach to pain management, complementing other physiotherapy interventions such as manual therapy, exercise, and education.

Conditions Benefiting from PMR

1. Chronic Pain Syndromes: Conditions such as fibromyalgia, chronic lower back pain, and osteoarthritis can benefit from the regular practice of PMR.

2. Postural Pain: Patients with pain from poor posture, such as forward head posture or rounded shoulders, may find relief through PMR as it helps reduce muscle tension and improve posture.

3. Tension Headaches and Migraines: PMR can effectively reduce the frequency and severity of tension headaches and migraines by decreasing muscle tension in the neck and shoulders.

4. Stress-Related Pain: Individuals experiencing pain exacerbated by stress and anxiety can benefit from the relaxation and stress-reducing effects of PMR.

Benefits of PMR in Pain Management

Physiological Benefits

1. Muscle Relaxation: PMR directly targets muscle tension, helping to release tight muscles and reduce discomfort.

2. Improved Circulation: Relaxed muscles improve blood flow, which can help in the healing process and reduce pain.

3. Reduced Muscle Spasms: By promoting relaxation, PMR can help decrease the frequency and intensity of muscle spasms.

Psychological Benefits

1. Stress Reduction: PMR has a calming effect on the nervous system, reducing stress and anxiety levels, which can indirectly alleviate pain.

2. Enhanced Body Awareness: Patients become more attuned to the sensations in their bodies, helping them identify and manage areas of tension more effectively.

3. Improved Sleep: Relaxation techniques like PMR can improve sleep quality, which is crucial for pain management and overall health.

Implementation of PMR in Physiotherapy Practice

Initial Assessment

Before integrating PMR into a patient's treatment plan, physiotherapists should thoroughly assess its suitability. This includes evaluating the patient's pain, muscle tension, stress, and overall health status.

Education and Training

Physiotherapists should educate patients on the principles and benefits of PMR. Demonstrating the technique and guiding patients through the initial sessions can help them understand and practice PMR effectively.

Guided Sessions

Initially, the physiotherapist may guide PMR sessions in person or through recorded audio instructions. This helps patients learn the correct technique and develop confidence in practicing PMR independently.

Home Practice

Patients are encouraged to incorporate PMR into their daily routine. Providing them with resources such as written instructions, audio recordings, or mobile app recommendations can support their home practice.

Key Message:

Progressive Muscle Relaxation is a valuable pain management technique in the physiotherapy toolbox. By systematically reducing muscle tension and promoting relaxation, PMR can help alleviate pain, reduce stress, and improve the quality of life for patients with various musculoskeletal conditions. Integrating PMR into physiotherapy practice provides a holistic approach to pain management, addressing both the physical and psychological aspects of pain. As research and clinical practice continue to evolve, PMR remains a foundational technique for enhancing patient care and outcomes in physiotherapy.

JOHN'S TRANSFORMATION: OVERCOMING PAIN WITH PROGRESSIVE MUSCLE RELAXATION

John had always prided himself on his work ethic and dedication to his job as an office manager. However, years of long hours spent hunched over a desk began to take their toll. Despite maintaining a generally healthy lifestyle, John started to experience persistent lower back pain.

At first, it was a minor annoyance, but over time, the pain became a constant companion, making it difficult for him to concentrate at work and enjoy his hobbies. Desperate for relief, John decided to seek help from a physiotherapist.

John's physiotherapist, Iman, greeted him warmly as he entered her clinic for the first time. She listened attentively as he described his symptoms and daily routine. Noticing his slouched posture and the tension in his shoulders and lower back, Iman suspected that poor posture and high stress levels were major contributors to his chronic pain.

"We're going to start with a thorough assessment," Iman explained. "I want to get a complete picture of what's going on with your body and how we can best address your pain."

Iman used a combination of visual observation, palpation, and digital posture analysis to assess John's posture and identify areas of muscle tension. As she suspected, John had significant muscle imbalances, with his lower back muscles overworked and his deep abdominal muscles underactive.

"John, what you're experiencing is quite common," Iman began. "Your posture and stress levels are causing muscle imbalances and tension, contributing to lower back pain. But don't worry, we have a plan to help you."

Iman introduced John to Progressive Muscle Relaxation (PMR), which involves systematically tensing and relaxing different muscle groups to reduce tension and promote relaxation.

"By focusing on tensing and then relaxing your muscles, you can achieve a deeper state of relaxation and help alleviate some of that tension in your back," she explained.

Iman and John formulated a comprehensive treatment plan that included PMR, ergonomic education, body mechanics training, manual therapy, and tailored exercises. Iman emphasized that addressing posture and muscle imbalances would be key to John's recovery.

1. Ergonomic Education: Iman helped John set up his workstation to promote better posture. He adjusted his chair height, positioned his computer screen at eye level, and used a lumbar support cushion. These changes made a noticeable difference in how he felt throughout the day.

2. Body Mechanics Training: Iman taught John how to perform daily activities, like lifting objects and sitting, in ways that minimized strain on his body. John practiced these techniques diligently, noticing gradual improvements in his posture.

3. Manual Therapy: Iman used joint mobilizations and soft tissue massage to alleviate muscle tension and improve alignment. Myofascial release techniques targeted the fascia, reducing pain and enhancing mobility. John found these sessions incredibly relaxing and felt immediate relief.

4. Exercise Prescription: John followed a tailored exercise programme designed to strengthen his weak muscles, stretch tight ones, and improve overall flexibility and alignment. He performed core strengthening exercises like planks and bridges and stretched his hamstrings and hip flexors. These exercises quickly became a part of his daily routine.

5. Progressive Muscle Relaxation (PMR): Iman guided John through PMR exercises during their sessions. They started with deep breathing to enhance relaxation, then systematically tensed and relaxed various muscle groups, from his feet to his head. John was amazed at how effectively this simple technique reduced muscle tension and stress.

John committed to practicing PMR daily at home, using an audio recording provided by Iman. He found a quiet place to sit, took slow, deep breaths, and followed the guided instructions. Each session left him feeling more relaxed and In control of his pain.

As weeks passed, John began to notice significant improvements. His pain behaviours diminished, and he no longer grimaced with every movement. His lower back ache subsided, and he felt more balanced and energized.

Iman shared two case studies with John one day to illustrate his progress. The first involved a 45-year-old office worker with chronic lower back pain, similar to John's situation. The patient's treatment included ergonomic education, core strengthening exercises, and manual therapy, resulting in substantial improvements. The second case was a 30-year-old with frequent headaches and neck pain who benefited from postural correction exercises, neck muscle stretches, and relaxation techniques.

John's journey highlighted the importance of understanding the relationship between posture and pain behaviours for effective physiotherapy intervention. By addressing his postural issues and modifying his pain behaviours, John significantly reduced his pain and improved his quality of life. He felt empowered by the education and behavioural modifications he had learned, leading to sustainable long-term outcomes.

John's story is a testament to the power of physiotherapy in transforming lives through optimizing musculoskeletal health. Through commitment, education, and the right techniques, he found relief from his pain and regained control over his body and well-being.

Reflection Exercise

Reflecting on John's journey to pain relief through Progressive Muscle Relaxation provides valuable insights for patients and health providers. These reflective exercises encourage deep thinking and actionable strategies for optimal pain management and physiotherapy outcomes. Use the following questions and prompts to guide your reflection, and write your responses in the provided space or a separate document.

For Patients:

1.   Think about your own daily posture. How does it compare to John's initial posture before he sought help? Do you notice any similarities or differences in how you feel?

Response: _____

_____

_____

2.   Reflect on the concept of Progressive Muscle Relaxation (PMR). How could this technique help manage your stress and muscle tension?

Response: _____

_____

_____

3.   John committed to daily PMR practice and other changes to improve his posture and reduce pain. What steps can you take to improve your posture and musculoskeletal health?

Response: _____

_____

_____

4. Identify any potential obstacles that might prevent you from practicing PMR or making ergonomic environmental changes. How can you overcome these challenges?

Response: _____

_____

_____

For Health Providers:

5. Reflect on how Iman assessed John's posture and pain behaviours. How do you assess similar cases in your practice? Are there any new techniques or tools you could incorporate?

Response: _____

_____

_____

6. Reflect on how you monitor and evaluate the progress of your patients. How did Iman track John's improvements, and what methods can you use to track your patient's progress?

Response: _____

_____

_____

Idea: Create a personalized health journal to document your daily posture, pain levels, and relaxation practices, including Progressive Muscle Relaxation (PMR). For patients, note typical postures and associated discomfort and record the effects of PMR on pain and stress. For health providers, include patient assessments, treatment plans, and progress observations. Reflect weekly to identify patterns and improvements. This journal will help you understand and manage posture and pain effectively, guiding both self-assessment and professional development.

C H A P T E R   9

PACING IN PHYSICAL REHABILITATION FOR PAIN MANAGEMENT

"Pacing is not about doing less; it's about doing smart. It helps patients sustain their rehabilitation efforts and gradually build their endurance and functionality."

-Dr. Sarah Wilson

Synopsis: *Pain management is a multifaceted endeavour that often requires a combination of strategies to address its various dimensions. One such strategy that plays a crucial role in physical rehabilitation is pacing. Pacing refers to the practice of balancing activity and rest to manage pain and increase functionality. In this chapter, we delve into the concept of pacing, its principles, and its application in physical rehabilitation for pain management.*

UNDERSTANDING PACING

Pacing is rooted in the recognition that chronic pain can disrupt an individual's ability to engage in daily activities. It involves breaking down tasks into manageable components and allocating appropriate periods of activity and rest to prevent the exacerbation of symptoms. The goal of pacing is not to avoid activity altogether but rather to find a sustainable rhythm that allows individuals to gradually increase their tolerance for activity while minimizing pain flare-ups.

(Andrews NE, 2015) discusses the concept of overactivity in individuals with chronic pain, where excessive activity can worsen pain levels, termed habitual overactivity behaviour. Activity pacing targets this behaviour, a common pain management strategy. However, empirical research on overactivity is limited. Andrews' study aimed to validate overactivity by correlating self-reported habitual overactivity with pain patterns, objectively measured physical activity, and daily activity participation in adults with chronic pain. Results supported the existence of habitual overactivity and its association with pain and activity patterns. Participants with high habitual overactivity levels but low activity avoidance were more likely to experience severe pain exacerbations due to activity engagement. This study provides initial support for overactivity as a legitimate construct in chronic pain. It suggests potential clinical applications for understanding and managing pain exacerbations related to activity. Andrews also hints at future research projects aimed at aiding clinicians in interpreting activity-related data for better pain management.

(Woznowski-Vu, et al., 2019) Conducted a study to address the inadequately assessed issue of increasing pain during physical activity in individuals with chronic musculoskeletal pain. They developed clinical measures called sensitivity to physical activity (SPA) indices to evaluate pain changes during brief physical tasks, employing three strategies: self-paced, standardized, and tailored. Their cross-sectional study involved 116 adults with chronic musculoskeletal pain and employed questionnaires, quantitative sensory testing, and SPA measures. Results showed that the tailored SPA index was most effective at evoking activity-related pain and uniquely associated with temporal summation of pain. It also served as a unique predictor of pain and pain-related interference, even when considering established psychological and sensory risk factors. This study underscores SPA as a crucial aspect of pain experience and highlights the value of using a tailored approach to assess it.

PRINCIPLES OF PACING

1. Gradual Progression: Pacing emphasizes gradual progression, starting with activities that are well within an individual's current capabilities and gradually increasing intensity or duration over time. This approach prevents overexertion and minimizes setback risk.

2. Activity Modification: Pacing involves modifying activities to make them more manageable and less likely to trigger pain. This may include breaking tasks into smaller steps, using adaptive equipment, or changing body mechanics to reduce strain on affected areas.

3. Scheduled Rest Breaks: Scheduled rest breaks are integral to pace. By incorporating regular periods of rest into daily routines, individuals can

prevent fatigue and pain from accumulating to intolerable levels. Rest breaks allow the body time to recover and recharge, improving overall endurance.

4. Mindful Awareness: Mindful awareness of one's body and its signals is essential for pacing. Individuals learn to recognize early signs of pain or fatigue and adjust their activity levels accordingly. This self-awareness empowers individuals to take control of their pain management and make informed decisions about when to push through discomfort and when to rest.

5. Flexibility: Pacing requires flexibility and adaptability. Plans may need to be adjusted based on changes in symptoms, energy levels, or external factors. Flexibility allows individuals to maintain a balanced approach to activity and rest even in the face of unforeseen challenges.

Application in Physical Rehabilitation

In physical rehabilitation settings, pacing is incorporated into comprehensive treatment plans aimed at improving function and reducing pain. Physical therapists work closely with patients to develop personalized pacing strategies tailored to their unique needs and goals. These strategies may include:

- Activity Grading: Breaking down rehabilitation exercises into smaller, more manageable tasks and gradually increasing difficulty as tolerance improves.

- Interval Training: Structuring physical rehabilitation sessions into alternating periods of activity and rest to prevent overexertion and optimize recovery.

- Goal Setting: Collaboratively setting realistic short-term and long-term goals to guide rehabilitation efforts and track progress over time.

- Education and Empowerment: Providing education about pacing principles and techniques empowers patients to take an active role in their recovery journey. Understanding how pacing can help manage pain and fatigue allows patients to make informed decisions about their daily activities and self-care practices.

- Monitoring and Adjustment: Regular monitoring of progress allows timely adjustments to pacing strategies as needed. Physical therapists can provide guidance and support to help patients navigate challenges and maintain momentum toward their physical rehabilitation goals.

Key Message:

Pacing is a fundamental component of physical rehabilitation for pain management. By balancing activity and rest, individuals can gradually increase their tolerance for activity, improve functionality, and reduce pain-related disability. Through careful application of pacing principles and ongoing support from healthcare professionals, patients can reclaim control over their lives. This will enable them to achieve meaningful improvements in their quality of life.

ECHOES OF RESILIENCE: A JOURNEY OF HEALING THROUGH PACING

In the bustling metropolis of Urbania, where life rhythm pulsed through every street corner and skyscraper, there existed a hidden sanctuary—a haven of healing nestled amidst the towering structures and bustling crowds. This sanctuary bore the name of Pacing Physical Rehabilitation Center, a place where stories of resilience and renewal unfolded like delicate petals unfurling under the gentle caress of the sun.

At the heart of this sanctuary was Alex, a once-vibrant soul now shackled by the chains of chronic pain. Once an avid adventurer, Alex found himself confined to the confines of his own body, dreams of exploration and excitement eclipsed by the shadow of disability.

Enter Harper, a physical therapist, a figure as revered as the ancient sages, whose presence brought a sense of calm amidst the storm of uncertainty. With a wealth of experience and a heart overflowing with compassion, Harper became more than just a physical therapist to Alex—they became a guiding light, a beacon of hope in the darkest of nights.

Together, they embarked on a journey—a quest for healing and restoration. But this journey was no ordinary one; it was a voyage into the depths of pain and perseverance, guided by pacing principles.

Harper, with the wisdom of a sage, unveiled these principles to Alex like treasures hidden in the depths of a forgotten cavern. They spoke of the art of gradual progression, where each step forward was a triumph, no matter how small. They delved into the intricacies of activity modification, teaching Alex how to reshape his world to fit the contours of his capabilities.

Scheduled rest breaks became interludes in their symphony of healing—a chance for Alex to pause, to breathe, to recharge. Mindful awareness became their compass, guiding them through the labyrinth of chronic pain and fatigue and empowering them to navigate the twists and turns of their journey with grace and resilience.

And yet, the road was not without its challenges. There were moments of doubt, of frustration, of despair. But with Harper by his side, Alex found the strength to persevere, push through the darkness and emerge into the light.

As days turned into weeks and weeks into months, Alex's journey became a tapestry—a mosaic of triumphs and setbacks, of highs and lows. But through it all, he never lost sight of the horizon, of the promise of a new dawn on the horizon.

And then, one day, as the sun painted the sky in hues of gold and crimson, Alex stood tall—a testament to the power of pace, to the resilience of the human spirit. With newfound vigour and a heart filled with gratitude, he embraced the world with open arms, his journey far from over but his spirit indomitable.

In the annals of Pacing Physical Rehabilitation Center, Alex's story became a legend—a beacon of hope for all who walked the path of chronic pain and perseverance. Harper continued to weave tales of healing, and his legacy was a testament to the transformative power of compassion and dedication.

And so, in the heart of Urbania, amidst the hustle and bustle of life, the tale of Alex and Harper echoed—a timeless reminder that within every challenge lies the seed of resilience and, within every journey, the promise of renewal.

Reflection Exercise

These reflective exercises are designed to deepen understanding, foster empathy, and promote effective strategies for managing chronic pain through the principles of pacing. Use the following questions and prompts to guide your reflection, and write your responses in the provided space or a separate document.

For Patients:

1. Reflect on the role of scheduled rest breaks in your daily routine. How do they help you manage your pain and energy levels? Describe a specific instance when a rest break made a difference.

Response: _____

_____

_____

2.   Imagine yourself in Alex's shoes. Visualize your own journey towards healing and renewal. What are the small triumphs you can celebrate along the way? How do you feel as you make progress, no matter how small?

Response: _____

_____

_____

3.   List three things you are grateful for in your journey of managing chronic pain. How has each of these things contributed to your resilience and ability to cope with challenges?

Response: _____

_____

_____

4.   Set a small, achievable goal for the next week that aligns with the principles of pacing. It could be a physical activity, a self-care practice, or a new hobby. Write down your goals and track your progress daily.

Response: _____

_____

_____

For Health Providers:

5.   Reflect on a patient you have worked with who, like Alex, faced significant challenges managing chronic pain. What strategies did you use to help them? How can the principles of pacing enhance your approach to patient care?

Response: _____

_____

_____

6.   Work together to set achievable goals for the patient's rehabilitation journey. Use the principles of pacing to break down these goals into manageable steps. Reflect on the process and how it strengthens the patient-provider partnership.

Response: _____

_____

_____

Idea: Patients and health providers can engage in a weekly Reflective Writing and Dialogue Session. Each participant writes briefly about their experiences related to pacing and healing, then shares their reflections in small groups. This fosters empathy, understanding, and collaborative problem-solving, helping both parties answer the reflective questions and strengthen their relationship.

CHAPTER 10

SUSTAINING PROGRESS: STRATEGIES FOR LONG-TERM SUCCESS

"Sustaining progress requires a balance of perseverance, adaptability, and a willingness to learn from setbacks."

-Dr. Laura King

Synopsis: In the annals of chronic pain management, the chapter dedicated to sustaining progress stands as a testament to resilience—a roadmap for navigating the winding path toward lasting wellness. Within these pages lie the strategies and insights gleaned from the collective wisdom of patients and healthcare professionals alike, each offering a unique perspective on the journey of healing.

It's crucial to establish a clear understanding of relapse for effective prevention and management strategies. While medical professionals typically define relapse as a return to an active disease state after a period of remission, particularly in chronic conditions.

Relapse encompasses a regression into dysfunction within the recovery process. It manifests itself as a progressive series of events that can lead individuals from stable recovery to dysfunction and, ultimately, back to dysfunction or other harmful behaviours. Recognizing this process is pivotal to early intervention and prevention.

Various factors contribute to relapse, including denial, stress, self-defeating behaviours, and social isolation. Those adopting a proactive approach to recovery actively manage obstacles and seek assistance when needed. Conversely, individuals prone to relapse may deny problems, leading to a downward spiral of coping mechanisms.

Relapse prevention planning is imperative across all healthcare domains, from chronic pain management to mental health treatment. It involves identifying high-risk situations and triggers, developing coping strategies, and establishing support networks. By addressing both the physical and psychological aspects of recovery, individuals can embark on a journey of self-discovery with optimism and appreciation.

(Cosio D, 2020) provides an insightful exploration into the intricacies of patient adherence and the prevention of relapse in chronic conditions. The article underscores the importance of understanding the distinction between "compliance" and "adherence," favouring the latter term due to its emphasis on the patient's active role in following a treatment plan over time.

The authors delve into various factors contributing to nonadherence, including demographic variables, attitudes, social support, and characteristics of the disease or injury. They advocate for a multivariate approach to addressing adherence issues, taking into account the patient-provider relationship, treatment regimen complexity, therapeutic environment, disease characteristics, client beliefs, patient characteristics, and social support.

The article discusses different measurement methods, such as self-reporting, behavioural indicators, biochemical indices, and clinical outcomes, to assess adherence. It emphasizes the importance of viewing adherence as a continuum rather than a binary concept. It suggests using multiple indicators to capture a comprehensive picture.

Furthermore, the authors offer evidence-based strategies for frontline and healthcare providers to enhance patient adherence and maintain long-term gains. These strategies include building a therapeutic alliance, employing motivational interviewing techniques, and utilizing health coaching interventions. They emphasize the shift towards a collaborative partnership between patients and providers, where mutual goals and shared decision-making drive treatment plans.

In conclusion, the article highlights the complexities of patient adherence and relapse prevention in chronic conditions. By understanding and addressing the various factors influencing adherence, frontline providers can optimize patient outcomes and promote long-term wellness.

Physical therapists play a crucial role in assisting individuals experiencing relapse or flare-ups in chronic conditions. Here are some ways we can help:

1. Assessment and Monitoring: Physical therapists can assess the current status of the patient's condition during a relapse or flare-up. They can monitor symptoms, functional limitations, and any changes in mobility or pain levels.

2. Tailored Treatment Plans: Based on the assessment, physical therapists can develop personalized treatment plans to address the specific needs of the patient during a relapse or flare-up. These plans may include modifications to exercises, pain management techniques, and strategies to improve mobility and function.

3. Education and Empowerment: Physical therapists can educate patients about their condition, the triggers for relapse or flare-ups, and strategies to manage symptoms effectively. Empowering patients with knowledge and self-management techniques can help them take an active role in their recovery process.

4. Exercise Prescription: Physical therapists can prescribe appropriate exercises to help patients maintain or improve mobility, strength, and flexibility during a relapse or flare-up. These exercises may be modified to accommodate changes in symptoms and functional abilities.

5. Manual Therapy: Hands-on techniques such as joint mobilization and soft tissue manipulation can help alleviate pain and improve mobility during a relapse or flare-up. Physical therapists skilled in manual therapy can provide targeted interventions to address specific areas of discomfort.

6. Modalities: Physical therapists can utilize modalities such as heat, cold, electrical stimulation, and ultrasound to manage pain and inflammation during a relapse or flare-up. These modalities can complement other treatment approaches and provide additional relief.

7. Functional Training: During a relapse or flare-up, physical therapists can focus on functional training to help patients perform activities of daily living with greater ease and efficiency. This may involve practicing specific movements or tasks relevant to the patient's daily life.

8. Collaboration with Healthcare Team: Physical therapists can collaborate with other members of the healthcare team, including physicians, psychologists, and occupational therapists, to ensure comprehensive care for patients experiencing relapse or flare-ups. This multidisciplinary approach can address the complex needs of the patient and promote holistic recovery.

By providing tailored interventions, education, and support, physical therapists can play a vital role in assisting individuals during relapse or flare-ups in chronic conditions, helping them manage symptoms effectively and improve their quality of life.

Patients can take several proactive steps to prevent relapse in chronic conditions:

1. Consistent Exercise Regimens:

Within the realm of chronic pain, exercise emerges as both a remedy and a shield—a potent tool for fortifying the body against the onslaught of discomfort. Here, patients discover the transformative power of consistency as they weave exercise into the fabric of their daily lives. From gentle stretches to targeted strength training, each movement serves as a testament to their commitment to progress. As they witness the gradual strengthening of muscles and the easing of tension, they find solace in the knowledge that resilience is not a destination but a journey—a journey that unfolds one step at a time.

2. Mindfulness and Stress Management Techniques:

In the sanctuary of mindfulness, patients find refuge from the storm of pain—a sanctuary where the cacophony of discomfort gives way to the serenity of the present moment. Here, they discover the art of letting go— the art of releasing tension and embracing tranquillity. Through mindfulness practices such as meditation, deep breathing, and guided imagery, they cultivate a sense of inner peace—a shield against the tumultuous currents of stress. With each breath, they reclaim a sense of control—a sense of agency in the face of adversity. And as they journey deeper into the realms of self-awareness, they emerge not as victims of pain but as masters of their own destinies.

3. Adherence to Treatment Plans:

Within the pages of their treatment plans, patients discover the blueprint for success—a roadmap that charts the course toward healing. Here, they find solace in the rhythm of routine—as they faithfully adhere to medication schedules, attend physical therapy sessions, and embrace lifestyle modifications with unwavering resolve. Through the trials and tribulations of daily life, they remain steadfast in their commitment to progress. They know that each pill swallowed and each exercise completed brings them one step closer to their goals. As they navigate the twists and turns of their journey, they find strength in the knowledge that they are not alone—that their healthcare team stands beside them, ready to offer guidance and support at every turn.

4. Education and Self-Empowerment:

In the halls of knowledge, patients discover the keys to their own liberation—the keys to unlocking a future free from the shackles of pain. Here, they delve into the depths of their condition, exploring its origins, manifestations, and potential treatments with a voracious hunger for understanding. Through patient education programs and support groups, they find solace in the company of others who share their struggles—a community bound together by a common quest for healing. And as they arm themselves with knowledge, they emerge not as passive recipients of care but as active participants in their own recovery—as architects of their own destiny.

5. Holistic Approach to Wellness:

Within the tapestry of holistic wellness, patients discover the interconnectedness of mind, body, and spirit—a truth as ancient as the earth itself. Here, they embrace the healing power of ancient traditions—from acupuncture to massage therapy to yoga—as they journey towards a state of balance and harmony. Through the gentle touch of a skilled practitioner, they feel the tension melt away—the knots of pain unravelling like threads in the wind. As they bask in the warmth of healing hands, they realize that wellness is not a destination but a journey—a journey that unfolds in quiet moments of reflection, nature's gentle embrace, and laughter shared with loved ones.

6. Ongoing Monitoring and Support:

In the embrace of their healthcare team, patients find solace in the knowledge that they are never alone—that their journey toward healing is supported by a network of dedicated professionals who stand beside them, ready to offer guidance and support at every turn. Here, they discover the power of collaboration—as they work hand-in-hand with their doctors, nurses, physical therapists, and counsellors to navigate the complexities of chronic pain management. Through regular check-ins, they find reassurance in the progress they've made—the milestones achieved, the obstacles overcome. And as they face the challenges that lie ahead, they do so with the knowledge that they are surrounded by a community of caring hearts—a community united in a shared quest for healing.

In the tapestry of chronic pain management, the chapter dedicated to sustaining progress is a testament to the resilience of the human spirit—a reminder that, even in the darkest of times, there is always hope. As patients embark on their journey towards lasting wellness, they do so with the knowledge that they are not alone—that, together, they will overcome every obstacle, scale every mountain, and emerge stronger on the other side.

JOURNEY BEYOND PAIN: SUSTAINING PROGRESS IN CHRONIC PAIN MANAGEMENT

In the heart of a bustling city, amidst the ceaseless rhythm of urban life, a sanctuary of healing and hope stood steadfast—a beacon of light amidst the tumultuous sea of existence. Serenity Haven Physical Rehabilitation Center, with its tranquil corridors and harmonious blend of medical innovation and natural serenity, serves as a refuge for those seeking solace and renewal.

At the epicentre of this haven was Maya, a spirited young woman whose once-vibrant life had been eclipsed by the relentless grip of chronic pain. Once a dreamer, her aspirations now seemed distant, shrouded in the haze of discomfort and uncertainty.

Yet within the walls of Serenity Haven, Maya discovered a glimmer of hope—a ray of light cutting through the darkness. Here, she encountered Lucas, a physical therapist, a beacon of compassion and understanding amidst the storm. With his gentle demeanour and unwavering support, Lucas became more than a physical therapist to Maya—he became her guide, her confidant, her champion in the battle for healing.

Together, Maya and Lucas embarked on a journey—a journey fraught with obstacles yet brimming with possibility. Theirs was a quest not merely to alleviate pain but to sustain the progress Maya had fought so tirelessly to achieve—to forge a path toward enduring wellness and vitality.

In the sun-drenched courtyard of Serenity Haven, Maya's journey to physical rehabilitation began. With Lucas as her steadfast companion, she embraced the transformative power of movement—a journey marked by determination, perseverance, and the occasional burst of laughter amidst sweat and tears. Through carefully curated exercise routines tailored to her individual needs, Maya sculpted her body and fortified her spirit, inching ever closer to reclaiming the life she once knew.

Mindfulness and Stress Management Techniques:

In the tranquil embrace of Serenity Haven's gardens, Maya found respite from the chaos of her inner turmoil. Under Lucas's gentle guidance, she delved into the practice of mindfulness—a journey of self-discovery and inner peace. Through meditation, graded motor imagery, deep breathing exercises, and the gentle embrace of nature, Maya learned to quiet the restless whispers of her mind, finding solace amidst the storm.

In the quiet sanctuary of her room, Maya pored over the intricate details of her treatment plan—a roadmap crafted with precision by Lucas and his team. With unwavering resolve, she committed herself to every aspect of her regimen—adhering diligently to medication schedules, attending physical therapy sessions with unwavering dedication, and embracing lifestyle modifications designed to nurture her journey toward healing. Through her unwavering commitment, Maya ensured that her progress remained steadfast, even in the face of adversity.

In the cozy confines of Serenity Haven's library, Maya embarked on a journey of enlightenment—a quest for knowledge that would empower her in her battle against chronic pain. With Lucas as her guide, she delved into the intricacies of her condition, seeking to understand its origins, manifestations, and potential treatments. Through patient education programs and the camaraderie of support groups, Maya found strength in the community—a network of fellow travellers united in their pursuit of healing.

In the nurturing embrace of Serenity Haven's holistic practitioners, Maya discovered the transformative power of ancient traditions. Through acupuncture, massage therapy, and the ancient art of yoga, she embarked on a journey of holistic wellness—a journey that nurtured her body, mind, and spirit in harmony. With each session, Maya felt the weight of her pain melt away, replaced by a sense of peace and tranquillity that resonated deep within her soul.

In the bustling corridors of Serenity Haven, Maya found reassurance in the presence of her dedicated healthcare team. With Lucas as her steadfast guide, she navigated the complexities of chronic pain management with confidence, secure in the knowledge that she was never alone on her journey. Through regular check-ins and the unwavering support of her caregivers, Maya felt a sense of reassurance that her progress was being monitored with care and compassion.

As the days turned into weeks and the weeks into months, Maya's journey toward healing continued unabated—a testament to the indomitable power of resilience and determination. As she gazed towards the horizon, she knew that with Lucas by her side and the unwavering support of her Serenity Haven Physical Rehabilitation Centre family, there was nothing she couldn't overcome. Together, they forged ahead, writing a new chapter in the story of resilience—one of hope, healing, and the triumph of the human spirit.

Reflection Exercise

This structured reflection and discussion exercise aims to enhance understanding, foster a supportive community, and develop effective strategies for sustaining long-term progress in chronic pain management. Use the following questions and prompts to guide your reflection, and write your responses in the provided space or a separate document.

For Patients:

1.   Reflect on a specific time when you felt a significant improvement in your pain levels. What actions or strategies do you think contributed to this improvement? How can you continue to incorporate these into your daily routine?

Response: _____

_____

_____

2.   Describe a challenge you faced in managing chronic pain and how you overcame it. What did you learn from this experience, and how can it help you in future situations?

Response: _____

_____

_____

3.   Consider your daily routine and lifestyle modifications. How have these changes helped you manage your chronic pain? What further adjustments can you make to sustain your progress?

Response: _____

_____

_____

For Health Providers:

4. Reflect on a patient's journey where they made significant progress. What specific strategies or interventions did you use, and how did they impact the patient's progress?

Response: _____

_____

_____

5. Think about the challenges you face in helping patients sustain long-term progress. What strategies have been most effective in overcoming these challenges, and how can you refine them further?

Response: _____

_____

_____

Idea: Pair patients with health providers for weekly one-to-one discussions focused on reflective questions. These personalized interactions foster deep connections and tailored support, enabling both parties to share insights and develop strategies for sustained progress and overcoming challenges. The buddy system enhances the healing journey and promotes long-term success through strong, empathetic relationships.

TAKING CONTROL: PHYSIOTHERAPY STRATEGIES FOR SELF-MANAGING PAIN

In the labyrinth of chronic pain, self-management emerges as a beacon of hope, offering individuals the tools and techniques to regain control over their lives. From a physiotherapy perspective, self-management is not merely a set of exercises or routines but a comprehensive approach encompassing physical, emotional, and educational strategies. This chapter delves into the multifaceted world of self-pain management, providing a roadmap to empower patients on their journey to pain relief and enhanced quality of life.

Understanding the Foundations

The first step in self-pain management is understanding the nature of chronic pain. Physiotherapists play a crucial role in educating patients about their condition, helping them differentiate between acute and chronic pain, and explaining the physiological and psychological aspects involved. This foundational knowledge equips patients with a better understanding of their bodies and the pain they experience, reducing fear and anxiety, which can exacerbate pain.

Goal Setting and Progress Tracking

Setting realistic, achievable goals is a cornerstone of effective pain management. Physiotherapists work with patients to establish short-term and long-term objectives tailored to their unique circumstances and capabilities. These goals serve as benchmarks for progress and motivation. Regular progress tracking through pain diaries or digital apps allows patients to visualize their improvements, identify patterns, and adjust their strategies as needed.

Exercise and Movement

Exercise is a pivotal component of self-pain management. Physiotherapists design personalized exercise programs that include stretching, strengthening, and aerobic activities. These exercises are chosen based on the patient's specific condition, pain levels, and overall health. Emphasis is placed on low-impact activities such as swimming, cycling, or walking, which improve cardiovascular health, muscle strength, and joint mobility without putting undue stress on the body.

Gradual progression is key to avoiding flare-ups. Patients are encouraged to start with manageable activities and gradually increase intensity and duration as their tolerance builds. Pacing, a critical strategy in chronic pain management, involves balancing activity with rest to prevent overexertion and subsequent pain exacerbations.

Stretching and Flexibility

Stretching exercises improve flexibility and reduce muscle tension, which can help alleviate pain. Physiotherapists guide patients through a series of gentle stretching exercises tailored to their needs. These exercises are designed to be performed daily and can be adjusted as flexibility improves. Regular stretching maintains joint range of motion and prevents stiffness, which is crucial for pain management.

Strengthening Exercises

Strengthening exercises target specific muscle groups to enhance their function and support the body's structure. Physiotherapists design these exercises to improve muscle strength without causing additional pain. Strengthening the core muscles, for example, can provide better support for the spine and reduce back pain. Gradual resistance training, using weights or resistance bands, is introduced as the patient's strength increases.

Aerobic Activity

Aerobic exercises, such as walking, swimming, or cycling, improve cardiovascular health and overall endurance. These activities also release endorphins, the body's natural painkillers, which can help reduce pain perception. Physiotherapists recommend starting with short durations and gradually increasing the time as endurance builds. Consistency is key, with regular aerobic activity being a crucial part of a long-term pain management plan.

Mindfulness and Relaxation Techniques

Chronic pain often has a significant psychological component. Mindfulness and relaxation techniques, such as meditation, deep breathing exercises, and progressive muscle relaxation, help patients manage stress and reduce the perception of pain. Physiotherapists guide patients in incorporating these practices into their daily routine, promoting mental and emotional well-being alongside physical health.

Mindfulness-based stress reduction (MBSR) programs have shown effectiveness in helping patients become more aware of their pain without being overwhelmed by it. By fostering a non-judgmental awareness of the present moment, patients can develop a healthier relationship with their pain, reducing its impact on their lives.

Meditation

Meditation involves focusing the mind to achieve a state of calm and clarity. Guided meditation sessions, often led by physiotherapists or trained practitioners, teach patients how to focus their attention away from pain and onto positive thoughts or neutral sensations. Regular meditation practice can help reduce anxiety and improve pain tolerance.

Deep Breathing Exercises

Deep breathing exercises promote relaxation and help reduce muscle tension. Techniques such as diaphragmatic breathing or paced breathing can be practiced anywhere and at any time, making them a convenient tool for pain management. Physiotherapists teach these techniques to ensure patients use the proper form and maximize benefits.

Progressive Muscle Relaxation

Progressive muscle relaxation involves tensing and then slowly releasing different muscle groups in the body. This practice helps patients become more aware of physical sensations and promotes relaxation. Physiotherapists guide patients through these exercises, which can be particularly helpful before bedtime to improve sleep quality.

Ergonomics and Lifestyle Modifications

Physiotherapists provide valuable advice on ergonomics and lifestyle modifications to minimize pain triggers in daily activities. This includes proper posture, ergonomic adjustments in the workplace, and safe techniques for lifting and carrying objects. Simple changes, such as adjusting the height of a computer monitor or using supportive footwear, can significantly reduce pain and prevent further injury.

Proper Posture

Maintaining proper posture is essential for reducing strain on the muscles and joints. Physiotherapists educate patients on how to sit, stand, and move correctly to avoid pain. Using ergonomic chairs, adjusting desk height, and taking regular breaks from sitting can all contribute to better posture and reduced pain.

Safe Lifting Techniques

Learning safe lifting techniques can prevent injuries and reduce pain. Physiotherapists teach patients to use their legs rather than their backs when lifting heavy objects, keep the object close to the body, and avoid twisting movements. These techniques are particularly important for individuals whose jobs involve manual labour.

Supportive Footwear

Wearing supportive footwear can make a significant difference in managing pain, particularly for those with lower limb pain or back pain. Physiotherapists recommend shoes with good arch support and cushioning to reduce the impact on joints during walking or standing.

Patients are also encouraged to integrate healthy habits into their lifestyle, such as maintaining a balanced diet, staying hydrated, and ensuring adequate sleep. These factors play a crucial role in overall pain management and recovery.

Heat and Cold Therapy

Heat and cold therapy are simple yet effective self-management techniques. Heat therapy, through warm baths, heating pads, or hot water bottles, helps relax muscles, reduce stiffness, and improve blood circulation. Cold therapy, using ice packs or cold compresses, is beneficial for reducing inflammation, swelling, and numbing sharp pain. Physiotherapists guide patients on when and how to use these therapies for optimal benefit.

Heat Therapy

Heat therapy is particularly effective for chronic pain conditions, such as arthritis or muscle stiffness. Applying heat can soothe aching muscles and improve blood flow to the affected area. Physiotherapists advise patients on the appropriate duration and frequency of heat application to avoid burns or overheating.

Cold Therapy

Cold therapy is beneficial for acute pain and inflammation, such as after an injury or during a pain flare-up. Applying cold can reduce swelling and numb the area, providing immediate pain relief. Physiotherapists guide patients on the safe use of ice packs or cold compresses, including the recommended duration and intervals to prevent skin damage.

Application of TENS Machine

Transcutaneous Electrical Nerve Stimulation (TENS) machines are a valuable tool in the physiotherapy arsenal for managing chronic pain. TENS machines work by sending small electrical impulses through electrodes placed on the skin. These impulses can help reduce pain signals going to the spinal cord and brain, relieving pain and relaxing muscles.

How TENS Machines Work

TENS therapy involves placing electrodes on the skin near the painful area. The machine sends electrical impulses that stimulate the nerves, which can block pain signals from reaching the brain. It also stimulates the production of endorphins, the body's natural painkillers. This dual mechanism can provide significant pain relief.

Using TENS Machines Safely

Physiotherapists educate patients on the proper use of TENS machines, including electrode placement, adjusting intensity settings, and determining appropriate duration and frequency of use. This knowledge empowers patients to use TENS therapy safely and effectively at home as part of their self-management strategy. Patients are instructed to start with the lowest intensity and gradually increase it to a comfortable level. They are also instructed to use the machine for no more than 30 minutes at a time unless otherwise advised.

Benefits of TENS Therapy

TENS therapy offers a non-invasive, drug-free option for pain management. It can be particularly beneficial for patients with chronic pain conditions such as arthritis, fibromyalgia, or neuropathy. By incorporating TENS therapy into their routine, patients can achieve additional pain relief, making it easier to engage in other therapeutic activities and maintain their daily functions.

Patient Education and Resources

Empowering patients with knowledge is a fundamental aspect of self-pain management. Physiotherapists provide educational resources, including pamphlets, videos, and online materials, covering various aspects of pain management. Topics may include understanding pain mechanisms, the importance of physical activity, and techniques for managing flare-ups.

Support groups and community resources also play a vital role. Connecting with others who share similar experiences can provide emotional support, practical advice, and a sense of community, all of which are invaluable in managing chronic pain.

Pain Education Programs

Physiotherapists often conduct pain education programs to help patients understand the nature of chronic pain. These programs may include workshops, seminars, or online courses covering topics such as the science of pain, pain perception, and effective self-management techniques. By demystifying pain, these programs reduce fear and empower patients to take an active role in their management.

Online Resources and Apps

There are numerous online resources and mobile apps designed to support pain management. Physiotherapists can recommend reputable websites, videos, and apps that provide exercises, mindfulness practices, pain-tracking tools, and educational content. These resources enable patients to access support and information anytime, reinforcing their self-management strategies.

Collaborative Approach

Effective self-pain management is a collaborative effort between the patient and the physiotherapist. Regular follow-up appointments

Key Message:

Self-pain management from a physiotherapy perspective is a holistic, patient-centred approach that empowers individuals to take an active role in their pain management journey. By combining education, personalized exercise programs, mindfulness practices, ergonomic adjustments, lifestyle modifications, and TENS therapy, physiotherapists equip patients with the tools they need to navigate the complexities of chronic pain. This collaborative, informed approach not only alleviates pain but also enhances the overall quality of life, fostering resilience and hope in the face of chronic pain.

FROM PAIN TO POWER: SAM'S JOURNEY OF SELF-PAIN MANAGEMENT

In the heart of a vibrant city, the Oasis of Healing Physical Rehabilitation Center stood as a sanctuary of healing. Its tranquil corridors and harmonious blend of medical innovation and natural serenity offered solace to those seeking renewal. Among the many individuals who found their way to this sanctuary was Sam, a spirited young man whose once-active life had been overshadowed by the relentless grip of chronic pain.

Sam had always been an adventurer, thriving on exploration and discovery. However, a severe accident left him with chronic pain that turned his dreams into distant memories. Day after day, he struggled with the physical and emotional weight of his condition, his aspirations obscured by a haze of discomfort and uncertainty.

At the Oasis of Healing, Sam met Luna, a compassionate and experienced physiotherapist. With her gentle demeanour and unwavering support, Luna became more than a therapist to Sam—she became his guide, confidant, and champion in the battle for healing.

Together, Sam and Luna embarked on a journey—a journey fraught with obstacles yet brimming with possibility. Luna began by helping Sam understand the nature of his chronic pain. She explained the physiological and psychological aspects, differentiating between acute and chronic pain. This foundational knowledge reduced Sam's fear and anxiety, empowering him with a better understanding of his condition.

The next step was setting realistic, achievable goals. Luna worked with Sam to establish short-term and long-term objectives tailored to his unique circumstances and capabilities. They tracked his progress through a digital app, allowing Sam to visualize his improvements, identify patterns, and adjust his strategies as needed.

Exercise became a pivotal component of Sam's self-pain management. Luna designed a personalized exercise program that included stretching, strengthening, and aerobic activities. They started with manageable activities, gradually increasing the intensity and duration as Sam's tolerance built. The pacing was crucial—balancing activity with rest to prevent overexertion and subsequent pain exacerbations.

In the sun-drenched courtyard of the Oasis of Healing, Sam began his physical rehabilitation. Through carefully curated exercise routines tailored to his individual needs, Sam sculpted his body and fortified his spirit. Gradual progression helped him avoid flare-ups, and each small triumph fueled his determination.

Chronic pain often has a significant psychological component, and Luna introduced Sam to mindfulness and relaxation techniques. Together, they practiced meditation, deep breathing exercises, and progressive muscle relaxation. These practices helped Sam manage stress and reduce the perception of pain, promoting mental and emotional well-being alongside physical health.

Sam embraced mindfulness-based stress reduction (MBSR) programs, learning to become more aware of his pain without being overwhelmed by it. By fostering a non-judgmental awareness of the present moment, he developed a healthier relationship with his pain, reducing its impact on his life.

Ergonomics and lifestyle modifications were also part of Sam's journey. Luna provided valuable advice on maintaining proper posture, making ergonomic adjustments in his workplace, and using safe techniques for lifting and carrying objects. Simple changes, such as adjusting the height of his computer monitor and using supportive footwear, significantly reduced his pain and prevented further injury.

Heat and cold therapy became simple yet effective tools in Sam's self-management strategy. Luna guided him on when and how to use these therapies—heat therapy through warm baths and heating pads to relax muscles and improve blood circulation, and cold therapy using ice packs to reduce inflammation and numb sharp pain.

One of the most transformative tools in Sam's self-management arsenal was the Transcutaneous Electrical Nerve Stimulation (TENS) machine. Luna taught him how to use the TENS machine, placing electrodes on his skin to send small electrical impulses that reduced pain signals to his brain and stimulated the production of endorphins. This non-invasive, drug-free option provided significant pain relief, making it easier for Sam to engage in other therapeutic activities and maintain his daily function.

Empowerment through knowledge was a fundamental aspect of Sam's journey. Luna provided educational resources, including pamphlets, videos, and online materials, covering various aspects of pain management. Sam attended pain education programs, workshops, and online courses to understand the science of pain, pain perception, and effective self-management techniques. This education reduced his fear and empowered him to take an active role in his pain management.

Support groups and community resources played a vital role in Sam's journey. Connecting with others who shared similar experiences provided emotional support, practical advice, and a sense of community, all of which were invaluable in managing his chronic pain.

Sam's journey was a collaborative effort between him and Luna. Regular follow-up appointments allowed for the assessment of progress, adjustment of treatment plans, and ongoing support. Open communication was encouraged, with Sam sharing his experiences, challenges, and successes, ensuring that his management plan remained dynamic and responsive to his needs.

As the days turned into weeks and the weeks into months, Sam's journey toward healing continued unabated. His story became a testament to the indomitable power of resilience and determination. With Luna by his side and the unwavering support of his Oasis for Healing family, Sam knew there was nothing he couldn't overcome.

One day, as the sun painted the sky in hues of gold and crimson, Sam stood tall—a testament to the power of self-pain management and the resilience of the human spirit. With newfound vigour and a heart filled with gratitude, he embraced the world with open arms, his journey far from over but his spirit indomitable.

In the bustling corridors of the Oasis of Healing, Sam's story echoed—a timeless reminder that within every challenge lies the seed of resilience and, within every journey, the promise of renewal.

Reflection Exercise

This structured reflection fosters self-awareness, empathy, and shared strategies for effective self-pain management through reflection on Sam's journey. Use the following questions and prompts to guide your reflection, and write your responses in the provided space or a separate document.

For Patients:

1.   Think about a specific technique or strategy you learned from your physiotherapist, similar to how Sam learned to use the TENS machine from Luna. How has incorporating this technique into your daily routine changed your experience of pain?

Response: _____

_____

_____

2.   Reflect on a setback you faced during your journey, much like the obstacles Sam encountered. How did you overcome it, and what did you learn from the experience that could help you handle future challenges?

Response: _____

_____

_____

For Health Providers:

3.   Reflect on a patient whose progress greatly improved under your guidance, similar to Sam's progress with Luna. What specific approaches or interventions did you use, and why were they effective?

Response: _____

_____

_____

4.   Consider the role of patient education in your practice, inspired by how Luna empowered Sam with knowledge. How do you ensure your patients understand and effectively apply self-management techniques? What improvements could you make?

Response: _____

_____

_____

Idea: Implement a weekly Guided Self-Reflection Program where patients and providers receive reflective prompts related to their pain management strategies. Participants can write in personal journals or share insights in an online forum. Optional monthly group meetings offer a space for discussion and support, encouraging regular self-assessment and continuous improvement in managing chronic pain.

PAIN SOLUTIONS

A STRATEGIC GUIDE TO MANAGING AND REDUCING PAIN

In the previous ten chapters, you have explored the fundamental aspects of understanding pain, including its various types, pathways, and impacts. You have learned to differentiate between multiple pain types: acute and chronic pain, nociceptive pain arising from tissue damage, neuropathic pain resulting from nerve damage, and centralized pain due to altered processing in the central nervous system. Furthermore, you have delved into the basic physiology of pain mechanisms, gaining an understanding of how pain is experienced and perceived. You have examined the significant effects of pain on physical function, mental health, and quality of life.

Physiotherapy plays a crucial role in managing pain through a holistic approach that addresses the physical, emotional, and psychological aspects of pain. You have also gained insights into evidence-based practices, emphasizing the importance of research-supported physiotherapy interventions in pain management. These practices underscore the value of using scientific evidence to guide clinical decisions, ensuring the most effective and efficient treatments for patients.

As we continue, we will build on this foundational knowledge to further enhance your understanding and application of effective pain management strategies. This next phase will integrate practical approaches and advanced techniques, equipping you with comprehensive tools to optimize patient outcomes and improve their overall well-being.

How to use this guide?

1. Consult Your Health Care Provider:

 - It's crucial to use this guide when consulting. They can offer personalized advice and adjustments to ensure the strategies align with your overall treatment plan.

- Regularly update your healthcare provider about your use of these strategies. This ongoing communication helps them track your progress and make necessary adjustments to your treatment.

2. Educate Yourself on Each Strategy:

- Take the time to thoroughly read this guide. Understanding each strategy is key to effectively managing your pain.

- Knowledge is power. By learning about different pain management techniques, you can decide which strategies may work best for you.

3. Assess Your Progress:

- Utilize the tools on the next pages to rate how well you do with each strategy. This visual tool provides a clear picture of your current status.

- Each phase represents a different strategy and is divided into four stages.

- Continue to use these tools regularly to track your progress. This ongoing assessment helps you identify areas of improvement and areas needing more focus.

4. Choose a Focus Strategy:

- Select one strategy that is particularly important to you and that you feel ready to start working on immediately.

- Choosing a strategy that resonates with you increases the likelihood of successful implementation and commitment.

5. Develop a Plan:

- Use this guile Action Plan provided on the next pages of this guide to develop a detailed plan for the chosen strategy.

- This plan should include specific, achievable goals and steps you can take to incorporate the strategy into your daily routine.

6. Experiment and Adjust:

- Begin implementing your plan and be prepared to adjust as needed. Many people find that their initial plan evolves as they see how it fits into their daily lives.

- Focus on starting with small, manageable changes rather than trying to perfect the plan before you begin. This approach allows for flexibility and reduces the pressure of perfection.

7. Monitor Changes:

- Pay close attention to any improvements in your ability to function and cope with pain. Note both small and large changes.

- Identifying which strategies provide the best results helps you refine your pain management plan and focus on the most effective techniques.

8. Keep Your Health Care Provider Updated:

- Regularly inform your healthcare provider about your activities, progress, and challenges.

- Their feedback and guidance are invaluable in ensuring your pain management plan remains effective and safe.

Four steps are suggested for effective pain management: Relief, Recovery, Rehabilitation, and Resilience.

<u>**Step 1: Relief**</u>

In this step, the focus shifts to the immediate alleviation of pain and discomfort through various pain relief techniques. These include the use of medications such as analgesics, paracetamol, and NSAIDs to manage mild to moderate pain. For more severe pain, prescription medications like opioids and muscle relaxants may be necessary.

Physical modalities also play a significant role in pain relief. Heat therapy, through warm packs, heating pads, or warm baths, can help soothe sore muscles and joints. Conversely, cold therapy, involving ice packs and cold compresses, effectively reduces inflammation and numbing pain.

Other methods include Transcutaneous Electrical Nerve Stimulation (TENS), which interrupts pain pathways to the brain, and massage techniques that relieve muscle tension and promote relaxation. Joint mobilizations, involving gentle movements, are used to improve joint function and reduce pain, contributing to a comprehensive approach to immediate pain relief.

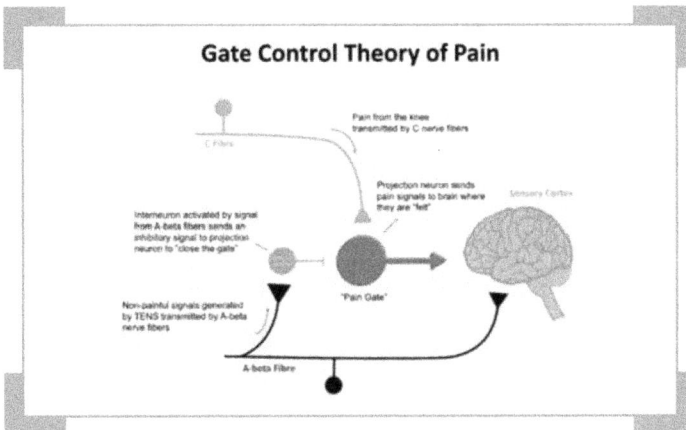

Gate Control Theory of Pain

Suggested Exercises for muscle tension and mobility

Stretching the neck may help a person relieve muscle tension and improve their range of motion. Below, we list examples of exercises that are best for pain with mobility deficits.

1. Chin Tuck

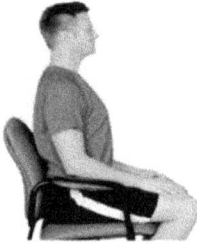

Sit with good posture   Tuck chin gently (nod yes)

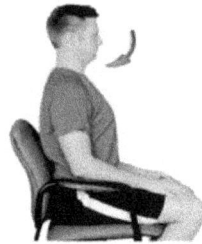

2. Cervical Retraction | Small Amplitude

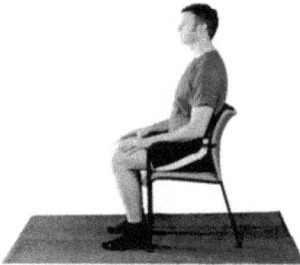

Sit in a chair with good posture   Gently tuck your chin as in nodding & Retract head slightly

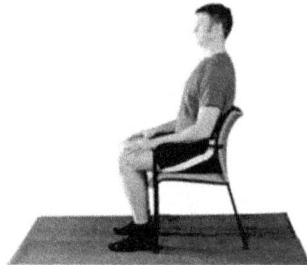

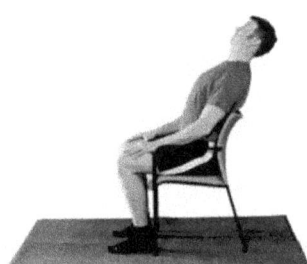

3. Cervical Retraction | Large Amplitude

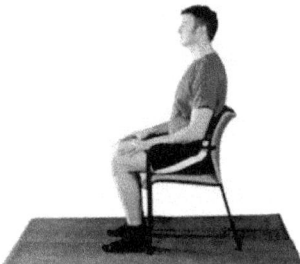

Sit in a chair with good posture   Gently tuck your chin as in nodding & Retract head

4. Chin Tuck + Trunk Extension (Chair)

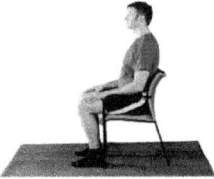

Sitting with chin tuck | Keeping chin tucked, back back | Arch over the lean of your chair

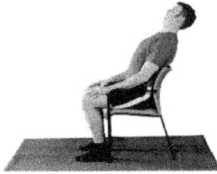

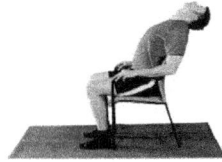

Guidance:

- Gently lower your chin as if nodding.

- Draw your head back and stretch your neck upward, looking towards the ceiling.

5. Cervical Segmental Rotation

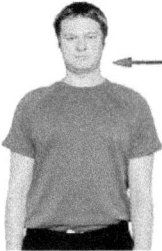

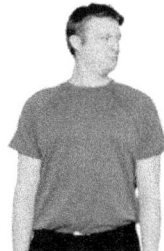

Tuck chin Maintain tuck, move slowly – Rotate head to side

Guidance:

- Gently tuck your chin as if nodding "yes."

- Slowly rotate your head to the side while keeping your chin tucked.

- Focus on moving smoothly from the top of your neck down to the base.

- Use a mirror to ensure you're not tilting your head to the side while rotating.

- Return to the starting position and repeat the movement in the opposite direction.

6. Cervical Segmental Flexion

Tuck chin   Maintain tuck, move slowly Continue to nod your head

Guidance:

- Maintain a good posture while sitting or standing.

- Gently tuck your chin as if nodding "yes."

- Slowly lower your head forward towards your chest, keeping the chin tucked.

- Focus on moving smoothly from the top of your neck down to the base.

- Return to the starting position with controlled movement.

7. Cervical Segmental Side flexion

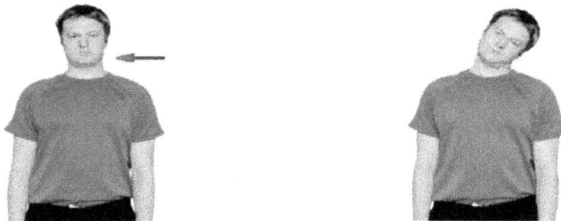

Tuck chin   Maintain tuck, move slowly -Bend neck to side

Guidance:

- Sit or stand with proper posture.

- Gently tuck your chin as if nodding "yes."

- Tilt your head to the side, bringing your ear toward your shoulder.

- Keep the chin tucked throughout the movement.

- Focus on moving smoothly from the top of your neck to the bottom.

- Use a mirror to ensure you're not rotating your head during the movement.

8. Shoulder Shrugs:

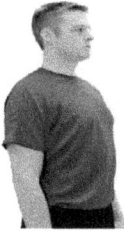

Stand tall, arms at sides   Raise shoulders to your ears.

Guidance:

- Stand upright with your arms at your sides, slightly in front of your body.

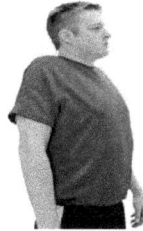

- Lift your shoulders towards your ears.

- Gently relax your shoulders back down.

9. Scapular Retraction:

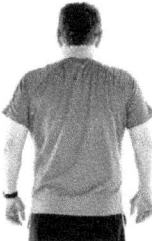

Stand tall with shoulders relaxed   Use muscles to squeeze your shoulder blades together and slightly downward; Head stays still

Guidance:

- Sit or stand with good posture

- It may be helpful to stand against a wall to feel the movement

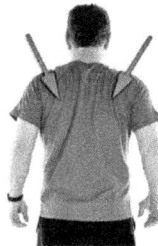

- Use the muscles between your shoulder blades to pull them together and slightly downward

- Be sure not to pull them together using your trapezius muscles (headache muscles)

- Relax and repeat

10. Scapular Clock

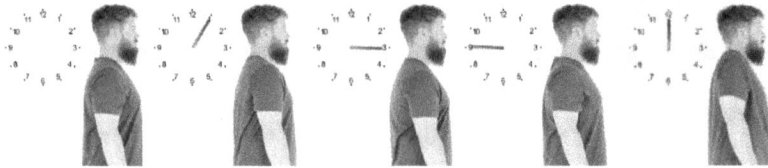

Start Position   Move shoulder blades to

1 o'clock   3 o'clock   9 o'clock   12 o'clock

Guidance:

- Stand tall with your arms positioned at your sides, slightly forward.

- Elevate your shoulders toward your ears.

- Gradually lower your shoulders back down in a relaxed manner.

- Move shoulder blades to 1 o'clock......3 o'clock... ...9 o'clock......12 o'clock, etc.

11. Thoracic Rotation

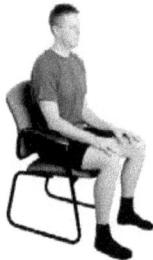

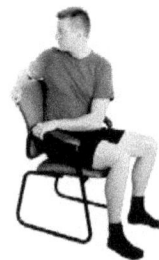

Start Position   Reach around the chair, pull the torso - avoid moving in the lower back

Guidance:

- Sit upright in a chair with proper posture.

- Wrap your arms around the chair as demonstrated.

- Gently twist your torso further.

- Experience a comfortable stretch in your upper back.

12. Repeat Trunk Flexion | to Floor

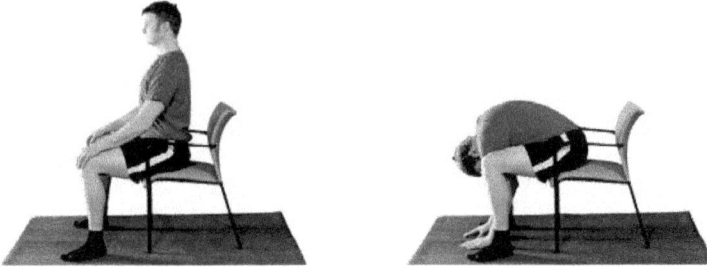

Guidance:

- Sit in a chair with proper posture.

- Place your hands on your thighs.

- Allow your torso to gradually lower toward the floor, using your arms to control the descent.

- Let your arms hang freely toward the floor.

- Then, use your arms to push yourself back up.

13. Lumbar Extension (Wall)

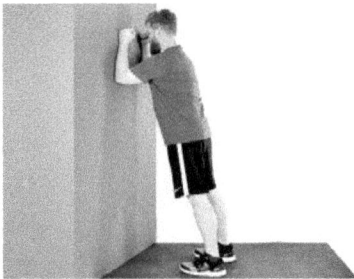

Start Position   Let hips sag forward -Hold - Repeat

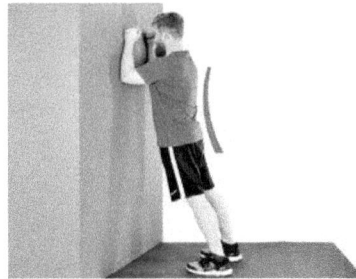

Guidance:

- Stand a few feet away from a wall, as demonstrated.

- Place your forearms on the wall for support.

- Allow your hips to sag forward and hold the position gently.

- Repeat the movement.

175

14. Gastrocs Stretch - Lumbar Neutral (Wall)

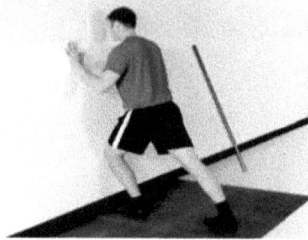

Keep your back heel on the ground to feel a stretch.

Guidance:

- Stand facing a wall, as illustrated.

- Prevent your lower back from arching by slightly leaning forward.

- Keep your back heel on the ground to feel the stretch.

15. Bridge

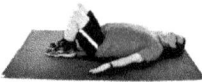

| Lie on back, arms resting at your side, palms up; Bend hips and knees, place feet on flat surface | Keep belly button pulled and squeeze glutes during movement | Lower slowly back to start position |

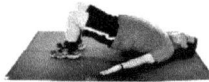

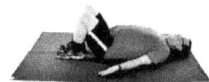

Guidance:

- Lie on your back with your arms relaxed at your sides, palms facing up.

- Bend your hips and knees, placing your feet flat on the surface.

- Engage your core by pulling your belly button in.

- Lift your hips off the surface to form a bridge, keeping your back from arching.

- Maintain the core engagement and squeeze your glutes throughout the movement.

- Lower your hips slowly back down.

16. Four Point Trunk Flexion + Extension

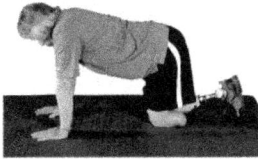

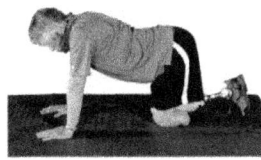

Go onto all fours   Arch back up   Arch back down

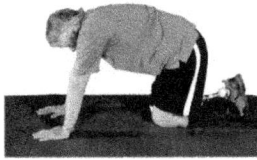

17. Lumbar Rotation AROM + Stretch

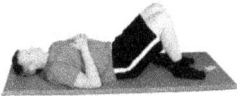

Start position   Roll to one side   Keep shoulder blades in contact with the floor

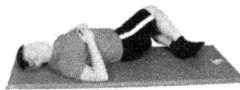

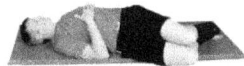

Guidance:

- Lie on your back with knees bent and feet flat on the floor.

- Gradually roll both knees to one side until you feel a stretch in the muscles along your side.

- Hold the position and take a deep breath.

- Slowly roll both knees to the other side.

18. Knees to Chest | Double Leg

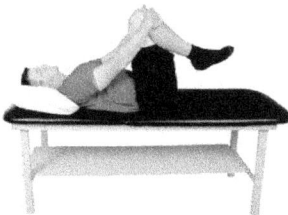

Wrap hands around   knees Pull knees to chest.

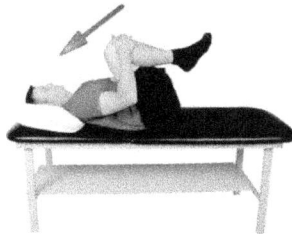

Guidance:

- Lie flat on your back with your knees bent.

- Bring both knees up toward your chest as far as possible.

- Wrap your arms around the front of your knees and gently pull, feeling the stretch.

- Relax and return to the starting position.

19. Repeated Lumbar Extension

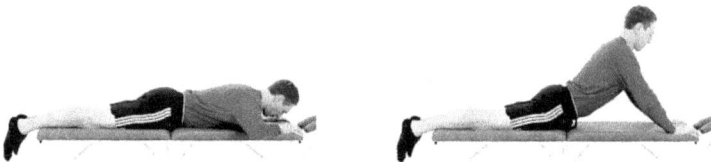

On Stomach   Sloppy push up

Guidance:

- Lie on your stomach with a pillow positioned under your hips.

- Execute a relaxed push-up by pressing your chest upward with your hands.

- Keep your hips resting on the pillow throughout the movement.

20. Repeated Lumbar Extension (Standing)

Start Position   Lean back

Guidance:

- Stand with proper posture, with your feet shoulder-width apart.

- Place your hands on the back of your hips.

- Gently lean back as far as you comfortably can.

- Slowly return to the starting position.

- Repeat the movement.

▪ Self-Help Strategies:

- Rest: Adequate rest periods are important to prevent overuse injuries.

- Relaxation Techniques: Breathing exercises, meditation, and progressive muscle relaxation.

21. Breathing exercise (Diaphragmatic)

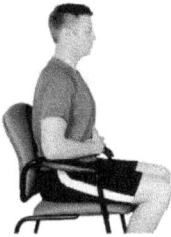

Hands-on stomach   Breathe stomach into hands

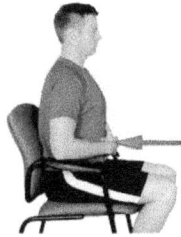

Guidance:

-        Place your hands on the front of your abdomen.

-        As you take a deep breath, allow your stomach to expand against your hands.

22. Meditation

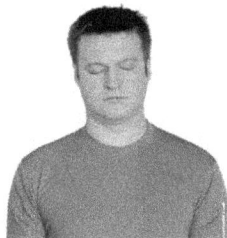

Guidance:

- Find a comfortable seated or lying position and relax.

- Begin to meditate.

Postural Adjustments:

- Ergonomics: Proper workstation setup, correct seating posture, and alignment during activities.

23. Posture Correction

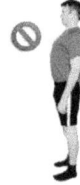

Slump posture   Correct   Avoid overcorrection

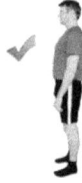

Guidance:

- Imagine a string gently pulling you upwards from the top of your head, allowing you to stand tall.
- Slightly lift your breastbone as you do this.
- Tuck your chin as if nodding 'yes' and hold the position.
- Gently draw your shoulder blades down and back.

24. Sitting Posture (Lumbar Roll)

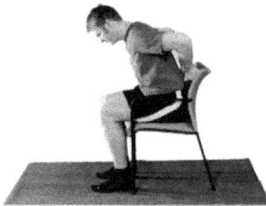

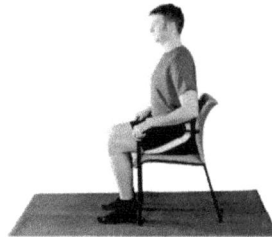

Guidance:

- Slide to the back of the chair.
- Place a roll behind your lower back.
- Sit up straight.

25. Posture (Desk)

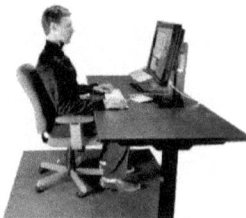

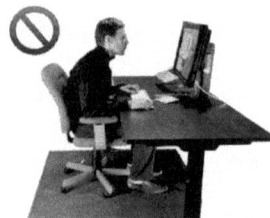

Good posture   Slouched- not good

Guidance:

- Select the right height for your adjustable desk or chair.
- Sit with proper posture.

26. Posture (Sit Stand Đesk)

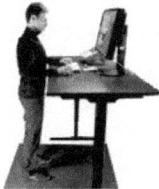

| Standing tall | Slumped- not good |

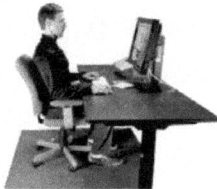

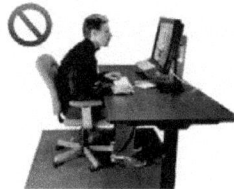

| Sitting Tall | Slouched- not good |

Guidance:

- Adjust your desk to the correct height.
- Stand with good posture.
- Sit with good posture.

27. Posture Standing (Stool, Desk)

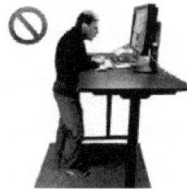

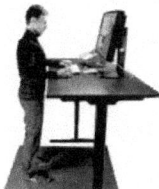

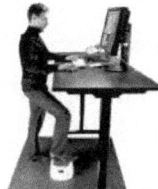

Guidance:

- Set your adjustable desk to the right height.
- Stand with good posture.
- To vary your stance, place one foot on a stool."

Posture is a widely discussed topic among patients, clinicians, the media, and society, with a common belief that spinal pain results from "incorrect" sitting, standing, or bending. Despite a lack of strong evidence supporting these beliefs, a large industry has emerged around posture correction products and interventions. Unfortunately, many healthcare professionals still offer advice based on these non-evidence-based views. An article published by The Journal of Orthopaedic & Sports Physical Therapy in July 2019 examines these common beliefs about posture and spinal health, explores why they persist, and discusses how clinicians can help reshape these misconceptions (Diane Slater, 2019).

Contrary to popular beliefs about posture, no substantial evidence supports the idea that a single "perfect" posture exists or that avoiding so-called "incorrect" postures can effectively prevent back pain. Spinal curvature naturally varies among individuals; no specific curvature is definitively linked to pain. It's important not to attribute pain to these relatively normal variations in spinal alignment (Wernli, 2022).

Posture can reveal much about a person's emotional state, thoughts, and body image. Sometimes, certain postures are adopted as a protective measure, reflecting concerns about bodily vulnerability. Understanding the underlying reasons for why someone prefers a particular posture can be valuable in addressing their overall well-being.

Furthermore, there is no evidence that postural and movement screenings effectively prevent pain in the workplace. People's preferred lifting techniques are often shaped by their unique spinal curvature, and there is no evidence to support the notion that adopting a specific posture or "bracing the core" benefits everyone.

Comfortable postures differ from person to person. Experimenting with various postures, including those that are often avoided, and making a conscious effort to change habitual postures might relieve symptoms for some individuals. Self-reported postural awareness is associated with clinical symptoms in chronic pain patients; improvements in postural awareness are longitudinally associated with reduced pain in patients with spinal or shoulder pain (Cramer H, 2018).

Example of Sleeping Positions: Recommendations for supportive pillows and mattress choices.

28. Cervical Sleeping Posture (Sidelying)

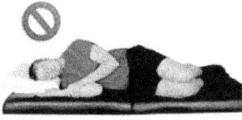

Insufficient support causes the neck to drop below the midline.

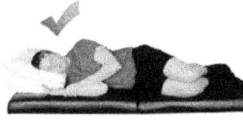

Neck neutral

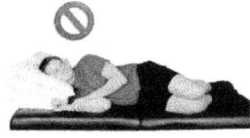

Neck positioned too high.

Guidance:

Proper sleeping posture is crucial to prevent your muscles and joints from being subjected to prolonged stress during the night.

29. Cervical Sleeping Posture (Sidelying - Pillow at Knees)

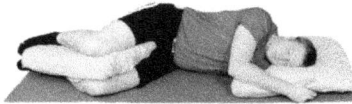

Sleeping position - pillow between knees

Guidance:

- Place a small pillow or cushion between your legs

30. Shoulder Sleeping Posture Sidelying

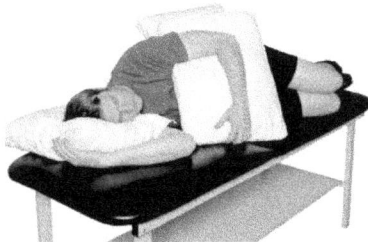

Position pillows as shown

Guidance:

- Avoid sleeping or rolling onto your affected shoulder at this time, as it is not recommended. The following position is ideal for resting your shoulder and should provide the most comfort.

- Lie on your side.

- Rest your affected arm on a pillow positioned from your stomach to your armpit.

- You may find it helpful to place your arm inside the pillowcase to keep the pillow secure while you sleep.

31. Shoulder Sleeping Posture Supine

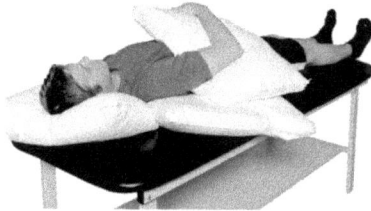

Position pillows as shown

Guidance:

- It's important to avoid sleeping or rolling onto your affected shoulder at this time. The following position is recommended to provide optimal comfort and rest for your shoulder.

- Lie on your back.

- Rest your affected arm on a pillow positioned from your stomach to your armpit.

- Consider placing your arm inside the pillowcase to help keep the pillow in place while you sleep.

- Place a pillow behind your affected shoulder to prevent rolling onto it during the night.

32. Lumbosacral Nerve Decompression

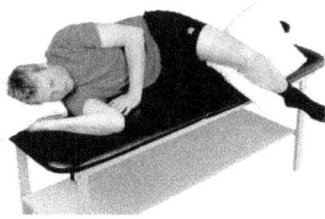

Front view

Guidance:

- Lie on your side with the affected side facing up.

- Place pillows between your knees.

- Slightly bend the affected hip towards your chest.

- Rotate the affected hip outward.

- Bend the affected knee over the pillows.

- Relax and focus on positive thoughts.

- Gently bend and straighten your knee.

- Gently pump your foot up and down.

- The focus is on nerve mobility, not stretching.

- Stop the exercise immediately if you experience any pins and needles, numbness, or tingling sensations.

33. Sidelying (Towel Roll, Pillow at Knees)

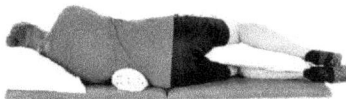

Position a rolled towel under your side and

place a pillow between your knees for support.

Guidance:

- Lie on your side, position a rolled towel beneath your side as demonstrated, place a pillow between your knees for support, and relax.

185

Pain management can be enhanced through various tools designed to support and reduce strain on the body. For instance, knee braces, back supports, and ergonomic tools effectively minimize pressure on joints and muscles, helping to alleviate discomfort. Additionally, assistive devices such as canes, walkers, walking poles, and orthotics play a crucial role in maintaining mobility and offering the necessary support to ease movement, thereby contributing to overall pain relief and improved function and quality of life.

The Brain Determines When You Feel Pain

Pain isn't always straightforward; while a damaged or worn-out body part can sometimes trigger it, this isn't always the case. There are situations where the pain lingers even after the affected area has been repaired, and in some instances, pain can occur without any apparent physical damage. The process begins when your body sends signals to the brain, which then interprets these signals, causing you to feel pain. However, it's important to understand that this communication isn't just one-way. The brain also can send signals back to your body, influencing the pain experience in complex ways.

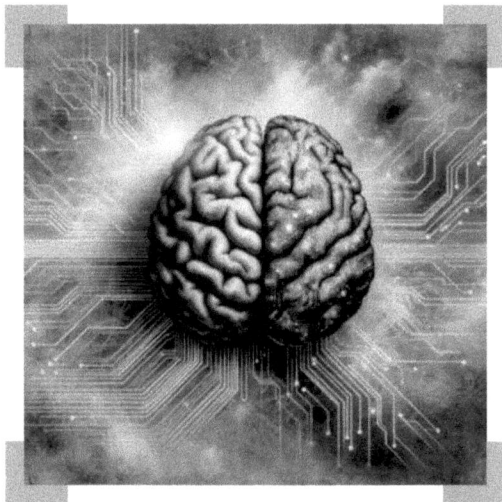

The Brain Controls the Opening and Closing of a Pain Gate

Managing pain effectively requires an understanding of the "pain gate" mechanism. When this gate is open, more pain signals reach the brain, intensifying the experience of pain. Various factors can lead to the gate being open. Emotional states such as depression, anger, and fear can heighten pain sensitivity. Negative or unhelpful thoughts exacerbate the discomfort, making pain feel more severe. Physical inactivity, like prolonged sitting, can also keep the gate open, while overexertion, such as standing or moving too much, can have a similar effect. Even pain medication, when used improperly or over long periods, can sometimes worsen the situation, particularly when it becomes less effective or is taken in higher doses than prescribed. Understanding these triggers is crucial for managing pain by keeping the gate as closed as possible.

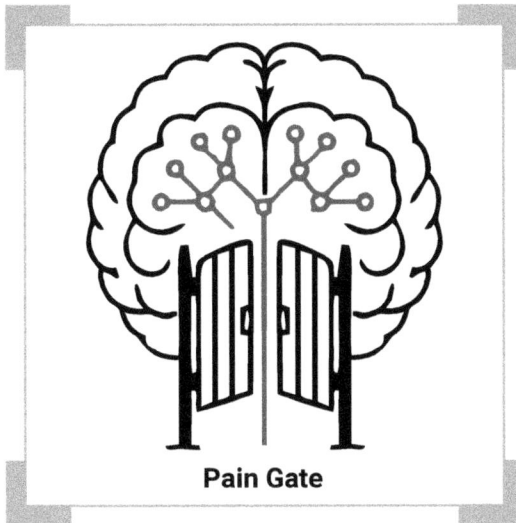

Pain Gate

Conversely, knowing how to close the "pain gate" is equally important in pain management. When done in moderation, regular physical activity can help maintain the gate's closure. Pacing your activities to avoid overexertion is essential. Cultivating a positive emotional and mental mindset can foster hope and significantly reduce pain perception. Additionally, when used correctly and under a doctor's supervision, pain medication can sometimes assist in closing the gate.

By combining these strategies—engaging in balanced physical activity, pacing oneself, fostering a positive outlook, and using medication appropriately—you can work toward keeping the pain gate closed, thereby minimizing the flow of pain signals to the brain.

Pain relief solutions can be optimized by utilizing various tools that support and reduce strain on the body, helping decrease your pain experience. Use the following tracking sheet to record which pain management modalities offer the most effective relief.

Pain Relief Technique used	Pain scale (0 -10) before (Pain location & intensity)	Pain scale (0 -10) after (Pain location & intensity)	Notes

Idea for Closing the Pain Gate:

1. Practice Relaxation: Set aside time to practice the Relaxation technique at least three times this week to help alleviate stress and promote relaxation.

2. Pace Your Activities: Focus on pacing yourself during physical activities at least three times this week, ensuring a balance between exertion and rest to manage your energy effectively.

3. Engage in Joyful Moments: Make it a point to do one small, pleasant activity at least three times this week to boost your mood and enhance your overall sense of well-being.

The Fear of Pain and Movement Can Become a Barrier for Physical Activity

Fear of pain and movement can often stand in the way of engaging in physical activity. Taking time to rest can be beneficial and support the healing process. However, if rest extends for too long, it can lead to additional problems, making it harder to regain strength and resume normal activities.

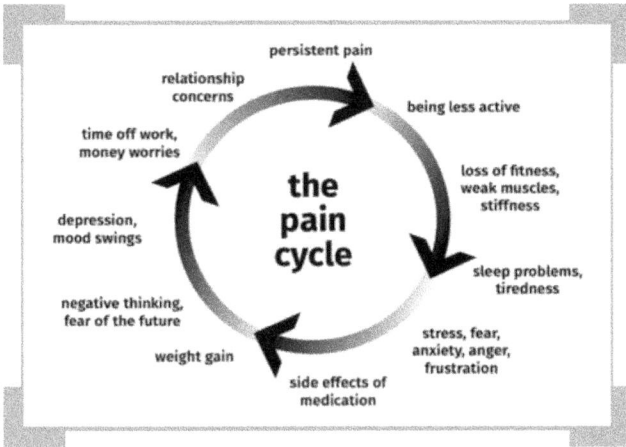

the pain cycle

persistent pain · being less active · loss of fitness, weak muscles, stiffness · sleep problems, tiredness · stress, fear, anxiety, anger, frustration · side effects of medication · weight gain · negative thinking, fear of the future · depression, mood swings · time off work, money worries · relationship concerns

Engaging in physical activity offers numerous benefits. It strengthens muscles, which act as a protective shield by stabilizing our bones and joints, helping us maintain balance and reducing the risk of pain. Strong muscles are crucial because weak ones can lead to increased pain due to their inability to support the skeletal system properly. Additionally, regular exercise can boost mood, potentially lessen pain, and distract from discomfort. It also promotes a sense of well-being and helps combat depression.

However, physical activity does come with some challenges. Finding the time and motivation to get started can be difficult, and exercise can sometimes lead to soreness. Overexertion, especially when doing too much at once, can trigger the pain gate, potentially increasing pain instead of relieving it. Balancing the pros and cons is essential to maximize physical activity while managing its potential drawbacks.

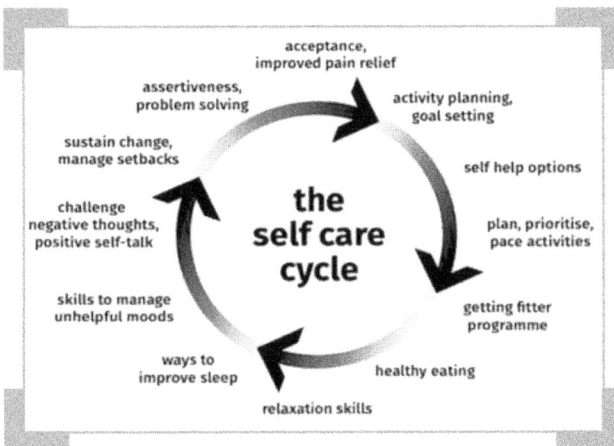

the self care cycle

acceptance, improved pain relief · activity planning, goal setting · self help options · plan, prioritise, pace activities · getting fitter programme · healthy eating · relaxation skills · ways to improve sleep · skills to manage unhelpful moods · challenge negative thoughts, positive self-talk · sustain change, manage setbacks · assertiveness, problem solving

Pacing your physical activities is an effective strategy to help manage and reduce pain by "closing the pain gate." Pacing involves striking a careful balance between activity and rest, allowing you to stay active without overexerting yourself. To effectively pace your physical activity, start by choosing something simple and manageable. Break the activity into smaller, more manageable chunks—perform one small part, then take a break. It's important to regularly check in with how your body feels. If you feel good after a brief rest, you can continue with another part of the activity. However, if you don't feel well, take additional time to rest before attempting more. Consistency is key; try to repeat the same routine each day for at least a week. If you need to reduce your activity on certain days, that's perfectly fine—just aim to return to your original goal when you're able. Gradually increase your activity level over time, paying close attention to how your body responds. If you find yourself wanting variety, consider switching to a different activity to keep your routine engaging. For more detailed information on pacing principles, refer to Chapter 9. Additionally, you can use the exercise tracking sheet table in the recovery stage to help structure your pacing plan.

Step 2: Recovery

The Recovery step is a comprehensive and multifaceted process to restore an individual to a state of health, normal function, and strength after experiencing an injury or illness. This process is not just about physical healing but also encompasses mental and emotional well-being, ensuring that the individual can return to their daily activities with confidence and resilience. Recovery is generally broken down into distinct phases, each with specific objectives and tailored interventions that guide the person from the initial injury to full rehabilitation.

Phases of Recovery:

1. Acute Phase:

Inflammation Control: During the acute phase, the body's immediate response to injury is inflammation, which, while essential for healing, can cause pain and swelling. Managing this inflammation is critical to prevent further damage and to set the stage for effective recovery. The R.I.C.E. method—Rest, Ice, Compression, and Elevation—is a widely used approach.

Rest allows the injured area to heal without additional strain.

Ice reduces swelling and numbs the area, alleviating pain.

Compression helps limit swelling and provides support to the affected area.

Elevation reduces blood flow to the injured area, further minimizing swelling.

Pain Management: Pain relief is a key component of this phase. Continuing the use of analgesics, NSAIDs (Nonsteroidal Anti-Inflammatory Drugs), and other medications prescribed during the relief phase ensures that the individual remains comfortable, which is crucial for both physical and mental recovery. Pain management at this stage not only alleviates discomfort but also prevents the pain from becoming chronic, which can complicate recovery.

2. Subacute Phase:

Mobility Exercises: As inflammation subsides, the focus shifts to restoring mobility. Gentle movements are introduced to regain the range of motion that may have been lost during the acute phase. These exercises are crucial for preventing stiffness and maintaining flexibility in the affected area. For example, if the injury is to a joint like a knee or shoulder, passive range of motion exercises might be initiated, where the joint is moved carefully within a pain-free range to prevent the buildup of scar tissue that could limit future mobility.

Gradual Activity Introduction: During the subacute phase, gradually reintroducing daily activities is important. This step is vital to avoid re-injury and to slowly build back the strength and endurance needed for normal life. The goal is to progressively increase activity levels while monitoring the body's response, ensuring that healing continues without setbacks. Activities are carefully selected and adjusted based on the individual's progress and pain levels.

3. Chronic Phase:

Strengthening Exercises: Once basic mobility and some degree of normal function have been restored, the chronic phase focuses on rebuilding strength. Progressive resistance training is introduced, gradually increasing the intensity of exercises to strengthen the muscles around the injured area and overall body strength. For example, if recovering from a knee injury, exercises might include leg presses, squats, and lunges, gradually increasing weight and resistance as the knee strengthens. This phase is crucial for restoring full function and preventing future injuries by ensuring that the muscles and joints are well-supported and capable of handling everyday stresses.

Endurance Training: Alongside strengthening, endurance training is introduced to improve cardiovascular health and stamina. This phase helps ensure that the body can sustain physical activity over longer periods without fatigue, which is important for returning to daily routines and, for some, athletic activities.

Activities like running, swimming, and cycling are common, with intensity gradually increased to match the individual's growing endurance.

Exercise Programs:

- Strengthening Exercises:

 - Core Stabilization: Core stabilization exercises such as planks, bridges, and exercises that target the abdominal and lower back muscles are critical for overall body stability. A strong core supports the spine, reduces re-injury risk, and enhances overall functional movement.

 - Targeted Strengthening: Specific exercises are designed to strengthen the injured area directly. For instance, exercises might include rotator cuff strengthening, shoulder presses, and rows if the injury was to the shoulder. These exercises ensure that the affected area regains strength and stability, which is key to long-term recovery.

- Flexibility Exercises:

 - Stretching Routines: Flexibility exercises involve dynamic (movement-based) and static (held positions) stretching routines. Dynamic stretches are useful in preparing the muscles for activity, while static stretches help to lengthen muscles and improve the range of motion after exercise. Flexibility prevents re-injury and maintains a healthy balance between strength and mobility.

 - Yoga and Pilates: Incorporating yoga and Pilates into the recovery process can significantly enhance flexibility and strength. These practices focus on controlled movements, breath control, and deep stretching, which benefit muscle recovery and overall well-being. They also improve body awareness, which helps in preventing future injuries.

- Cardiovascular Conditioning:

 - Low-Impact Activities: Low-impact exercises such as walking, swimming, and cycling are particularly beneficial during recovery as they provide cardiovascular benefits without placing undue stress on the injured area. These activities help maintain cardiovascular fitness, which is essential for overall health and endurance.

- Aerobic Exercises: Structured aerobic routines, which might include activities like running, brisk walking, or using an elliptical machine, are introduced as the individual progresses. These exercises improve heart health, boost energy levels, and support weight management, all contributing to a more robust recovery.

The optimum heart rate at which you should train for an effective workout is known as your "target heart rate zone." This zone represents the range of heartbeats per minute (bpm) that allows your body to benefit most from cardiovascular exercise, whether your goal is to improve cardiovascular health, burn fat, or enhance overall fitness.

How to Determine Your Target Heart Rate Zone?

1. Calculate Your Maximum Heart Rate (MHR):

- The maximum heart rate estimates the highest number of times your heart can beat per minute during maximum effort.

- A common formula to calculate MHR is `220 - your age = MHR`.

- For example, if you're 30 years old: `220 - 30 = 190 bpm` (This is your estimated MHR).

2. Determine Your Target Heart Rate Zone:

The American Heart Association generally recommends these heart rates:

- Your target heart rate is typically 50% to 70% of your MHR for moderate-intensity exercise.

- Your target heart rate is 70% to 85% of your MHR for vigorous-intensity exercise.

Here's how to calculate it:

- Lower end of the zone: MHR × 0.50 = lower end of target zone`

- Upper end of the zone: MHR × 0.85 = upper end of target zone`

Example:

- For a 30-year-old with an MHR of 190 bpm:

- Lower end: `190 × 0.50 = 95 bpm`

- Upper end: `190 × 0.85 = 161.5 bpm`

- So, the target heart rate zone for a 30-year-old is approximately 95 to 162 bpm.

Why Exercise Within the Target Heart Rate Zone?

1. Cardiovascular Fitness:

- Training within the target heart rate zone helps improve cardiovascular endurance by strengthening the heart and lungs.

2. Fat Burning:

- Exercising at a lower intensity (50-70% of MHR) is often recommended for fat burning, as your body primarily uses fat as fuel at this intensity.

3. Performance Improvement:

- Higher-intensity workouts (70-85% of MHR) are great for increasing aerobic capacity, endurance, and overall fitness levels.

4. Safety:

- Staying within your target heart rate zone helps prevent overtraining and reduces the risk of injury or burnout.

Monitoring Your Heart Rate

To ensure you're training within your target heart rate zone:

- Manual Check: Periodically check your pulse during exercise by counting your heartbeats for 15 seconds and multiplying by 4 to get bpm.

- Heart Rate Monitor: Wearable devices or fitness trackers can provide real-time monitoring, making staying within your target zone easier.

- Smartphone Apps: Many apps sync with heart rate monitors to track and analyze your heart rate data during workouts.

Adjustments Based on Fitness Level and Goals

- Beginners: Start at the lower end of your target heart rate zone (50-60% of MHR) and gradually increase the intensity as your fitness improves.

- Experienced Athletes: Training closer to the upper end of the zone (70-85% of MHR) can help improve speed, endurance, and overall athletic performance.

- Special Considerations: If you have any health conditions or are taking medications that affect your heart rate, consult with a healthcare provider before starting a new exercise regimen.

By training within your target heart rate zone, you can maximize the effectiveness of your workouts, whether your goal is to improve health, lose weight, or boost athletic performance.

Zone 1 (recovery/easy)	55%-65% HR max	Used to get your body moving with minimal stress and exertion. This zone might be used for an easy training day, warming up or cooling down.
Zone 2 (aerobic/base)	65%-75% HR max	Used for longer training sessions, you can sustain this basic-effort zone for many miles, yet still chitchat a little bit with your workout partner.
Zone 3 (tempo)	80%-85% HR max	This zone is where you push the pace to build up speed and strength; conversation is reduced to single words.
Zone 4 (lactate threshold)	85%-88% HR max	In this zone, your body is processing its maximum amount of lactic acid as a fuel source; above this level, lactic acid builds up too quickly to be processed and fatigues muscles; training in this zone helps your body develop efficiency when you're operating at your maximum sustainable pace.
Zone 5 (anaerobic)	90% HR max and above	This maximum speed zone (think closing kick in a race) trains the neuromuscular system—your body learns to recruit additional muscle fibers and fire muscles more effectively.

Adopted from www.rci.com

Choosing the Right Exercise Intensity for Pain Management

Effectively managing pain through exercise requires a carefully tailored approach, where exercise intensity is adjusted to match your needs, limitations, and the nature of your pain. Exercise can be a powerful tool in pain management, but only when applied thoughtfully. Below, I've outlined a set of guidelines that blend insights from my clinical experience with established professional exercise recommendations, specifically modified to address the unique challenges of pain management:

1. Start Low and Go Slow: Begin with low-intensity exercises to assess your body's response. Gradually increase the intensity as your tolerance improves. This helps avoid flare-ups and allows your body to adapt to new activity levels.

2. Listen to Your Body: Pay close attention to how your body responds during and after exercise. If you experience increased pain that persists beyond 24 hours, it may indicate that the intensity was too high, and adjustments are needed.

3. Incorporate Rest Days: Ensure that your exercise routine includes rest days to allow your body to recover. Overtraining can exacerbate pain and lead to setbacks in your pain management efforts.

4. Focus on Functionality: Prioritize exercises that improve your daily functionality and quality of life. Activities enhancing mobility, strength, and endurance can significantly reduce pain and overall well-being.

5. Modify as Needed: Don't hesitate to modify exercises to accommodate your pain levels or physical limitations. Adjusting the range of motion, duration, or resistance can make exercises more manageable and effective.

6. Consult with Professionals: Regularly consult with healthcare providers or physical therapists specializing in pain management. They can provide personalized guidance and help you navigate any challenges during your exercise program.

7. Stay Consistent: Consistency is key to seeing benefits in pain management. While it's important to avoid overdoing it, maintaining a regular exercise schedule can help gradually build strength and resilience, leading to better pain control over time.

By following these guidelines, you can create an exercise plan that helps manage your pain and supports your overall health and well-being.

Remember, the goal is to enhance your quality of life, so finding the right balance in exercise intensity is essential.

- Aerobic Activity: Aim for at least 150 minutes of moderate aerobic exercise per week or 75 minutes of vigorous activity if your condition allows. A mix of both can also be effective. Spread your exercise sessions throughout the week to avoid overloading your body. For additional benefits, particularly in managing chronic pain, try gradually increasing to 300 minutes of moderate aerobic activity weekly. Even short bursts of activity throughout the day can improve overall pain relief and function.

- Moderate Exercise for Pain Management includes gentle walking, stationary biking, swimming, or aquatic exercises, which are easier on the joints and muscles.

- Examples of Vigorous Exercise (if tolerated): Light jogging, water aerobics, or tailored aerobic dancing.

- Strength Training: Engage in strength training for all major muscle groups at least twice weekly, focusing on low-impact exercises. Start with one set per exercise, using a resistance level to complete 12 to 15 repetitions without exacerbating your pain. Strength training can help improve muscle support around painful areas, reducing discomfort.

- Examples for Pain Management: Resistance bands, light free weights, or body-weight exercises like modified squats, wall push-ups, or gentle planks. Activities like yoga or Pilates can also be beneficial for strengthening without straining.

When exercising for pain management, the intensity should be moderate, gradually increasing as your body adapts. Avoid pushing yourself too hard, as overexertion can worsen pain. Start with light intensity and build up slowly, aiming for a 5% to 10% increase in weekly activity. Always listen to your body and adjust as needed to avoid flare-ups (refer to the flare-ups plan included in this guide)

Focus on your goals—whether reducing pain, improving mobility, or enhancing overall well-being—to determine the right exercise intensity. Fitness and pain management are long-term commitments, so avoid rushing the process. Consult with a healthcare provider or physical therapist to create a safe, personalized exercise plan that considers your specific pain conditions.

IDRIS HAFIZ

Example of Exercise Tracking Sheet

Week #1	Baseline	Day 1	Day 2	Day 3	Day 4	Day 5	Day 6	Day 7
Example of exercise	in sec, min or reps/# of sessions							
Mini elliptical exercise	5 minutes 2x daily	5.2 minutes 2x daily	5.5 minutes 2x daily	5.7 minutes 2x daily	6 minutes 2x daily	6.2 minutes 2x daily	Rest	6.7 minutes 2x daily
6MI Exercise	2-3x daily	2-3x daily	2-3x daily	Rest	2-3x daily	2-3x daily	Rest	2-3x daily
Neck Range of Motion	8 reps 2x/daily all direction s	8 reps 2x/daily	8 reps 2x/daily	Rest	8 reps 2x/daily	8 reps 2x/daily	Rest	8 reps 2x/daily
Left knee extensio (ROM)	8 reps 2x/daily	8 reps 2x/daily	8 reps 2x/daily	Rest	8 reps 2x/daily	8 reps 2x/daily	8 reps 2x/daily	8 reps 2x/daily

Nutrition and Hydration:

Seek advice from a nutritionist or dietitian and refer to Chapter 6 of this book for further information on nutrition and managing chronic pain.

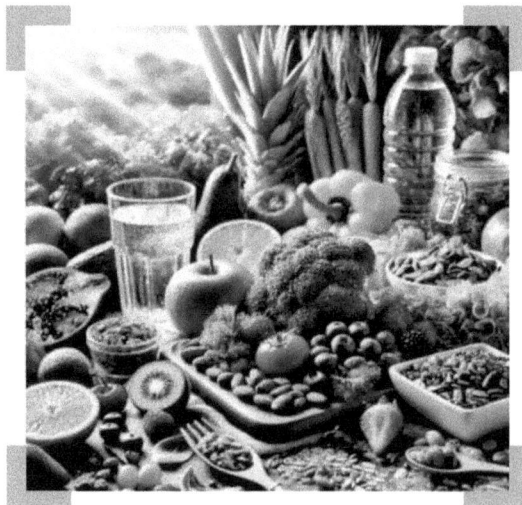

- Dietary Considerations:

- Anti-Inflammatory Foods: Diet plays a crucial role in the recovery process. Consuming foods rich in omega-3 fatty acids (found in fish like salmon and flaxseeds), antioxidants (found in berries, nuts, and leafy greens), and fiber (found in whole grains, fruits, and vegetables) can help reduce inflammation and support healing.

- Balanced Nutrition: A well-rounded diet that includes sufficient protein (for muscle repair), healthy fats (for cellular health), and carbohydrates (for energy) is essential. Proper nutrition supports physical recovery and mental well-being, providing the energy and nutrients needed for the body to heal efficiently.

Hydration:

- Water Intake: Staying hydrated is vital for maintaining muscle function, joint lubrication, and overall cellular health. Adequate water intake helps flush out toxins, reduce fatigue, and support every physiological process involved in recovery.

- Electrolytes: Particularly during physical activity, maintaining electrolyte balance is important. Electrolytes such as sodium, potassium, and magnesium are crucial for nerve function, muscle contractions, and overall hydration. Proper electrolyte balance ensures that the body functions optimally, especially during the more active phases of recovery.

In conclusion, the recovery process is a dynamic journey that requires careful attention to various factors, including pain management, exercise, nutrition, and hydration. Each phase builds on the previous one, ensuring that the individual progresses from injury to full recovery in a structured and effective manner. This holistic approach promotes physical healing and supports overall well-being, empowering individuals to regain their health, strength, and confidence.

Step 3: Rehabilitation

The rehabilitation step is a structured and comprehensive program designed to assist individuals in regaining their function, mobility, and strength following an injury, surgery, or chronic illness. This process is vital for restoring independence and improving the quality of life. The approach to rehabilitation is personalized, addressing the unique needs of each individual through targeted interventions and progressive strategies.

Individualized Rehabilitation Plans:

- Assessment and Goal Setting:

  - Initial Assessment: The rehabilitation process begins with a thorough initial assessment, where a healthcare professional comprehensively evaluates the patient's physical condition. This includes assessing pain levels, functional limitations, range of motion, muscle strength, and any specific challenges the individual may face in their daily activities. The assessment serves as the foundation for developing a tailored rehabilitation plan.

  - Goal Setting: Based on the initial assessment, specific goals are set to guide the rehabilitation process. These goals follow the SMART framework—Specific, Measurable, Achievable, Relevant, and Time-bound. Setting clear and realistic goals ensures that the patient and the healthcare team clearly understand the desired outcomes and can track progress over time. For example, a goal might be to regain a shoulder's full range of motion within six weeks or to walk independently for 30 minutes within three months.

- Progressive Exercises:

  - Gradual Intensity Increase: Rehabilitation exercises are designed to gradually increase in intensity as the patient's strength and mobility improve. Initially, the focus may be on basic movements and low-impact exercises to avoid overloading the injured or weakened area. As the patient progresses, more advanced exercises are introduced to build strength, endurance, and flexibility. This gradual progression helps in preventing re-injury and ensures sustainable improvement.

  - Functional Training: Functional training is a critical component of rehabilitation, emphasizing exercises that mimic daily activities. The goal is to restore practical functionality, enabling the patient to perform everyday tasks with ease and confidence. This may include exercises that simulate lifting, bending, walking, or climbing stairs, depending on the patient's specific needs and lifestyle.

Therapeutic Intervention

- Physical Therapy Modalities:

  - Hydrotherapy, or water-based exercises, is particularly beneficial for individuals with joint pain or mobility issues. The buoyancy of water reduces the stress on joints while providing resistance to build strength.

This makes hydrotherapy an excellent choice for those recovering from lower limb injuries or managing chronic conditions like arthritis.

- Electrotherapy involves using electrical currents to relieve pain, reduce inflammation, and stimulate muscle contractions. Techniques such as TENS (Transcutaneous Electrical Nerve Stimulation) are commonly used to manage pain, while other forms of electrotherapy can help in muscle re-education and recovery.

- Manual Therapy involves hands-on techniques a skilled therapist applies to manipulate and mobilize muscles, joints, and soft tissues. Advanced techniques such as myofascial release, which targets the fascia (connective tissue that surrounds muscles), and trigger point therapy, which focuses on relieving tension in specific areas, are used to alleviate pain, improve circulation, and enhance mobility.

- Occupational Therapy:

- Daily Living Skills: Occupational therapy focuses on helping individuals regain the ability to perform daily living tasks independently. This includes activities like dressing, bathing, cooking, and other essential functions. The therapist works with the patient to develop strategies and use adaptive equipment, if necessary, to improve their ability to manage these tasks.

- Work-Related Functions: Occupational therapy may include job-specific training for those returning to work after an injury or illness. This involves adapting tasks and work environments to ensure the patient can perform their duties safely and efficiently. The therapist may suggest ergonomic adjustments or provide strategies to reduce strain and prevent future injuries.

Patient Education

- *Self-Management Skills:*

- Home Exercise Programs: To ensure continuity of care, patients are often provided with home exercise programs. These programs are tailored to the individual's needs and designed to complement the in-clinic rehabilitation sessions. Regularly performing these exercises at home is crucial for maintaining progress and preventing regression.

- Pain Monitoring: Education on pain monitoring is an integral part of rehabilitation. Patients learn to recognize early signs of discomfort or pain and understand their triggers. This knowledge empowers them to take proactive steps in managing pain, whether through modifying activities, using pain relief techniques, or adjusting their exercise regimen.

- Preventive Strategies:

- <u>Preventing re-injury</u> is a key focus of rehabilitation. Patients are taught strategies to protect the injured area and reduce the risk of future injuries. This may include proper body mechanics, safe lifting techniques, and posture awareness during activities.

- <u>Healthy Habits:</u> Rehabilitation also emphasizes the importance of healthy lifestyle habits supporting long-term well-being. This includes regular physical activity, balanced nutrition, and adequate rest and sleep. These habits aid in recovery and contribute to overall health, reducing the likelihood of future injuries or health issues.

In summary, rehabilitation is a dynamic and individualized process beyond mere recovery. It involves a combination of personalized exercises, therapeutic interventions, patient education, and preventive strategies, all aimed at restoring the individual's physical capabilities and enhancing their quality of life. By focusing on both immediate recovery and long-term health, rehabilitation programs empower patients to regain their independence and confidently return to their daily routines.

Step 4: Resilience

In this final step, you will learn about building resilience in Pain Management. Resilience in the context of pain management is the ability to adapt to and recover from pain and setbacks while maintaining a positive outlook and continuing to make progress. It's about building the mental and emotional strength necessary to navigate the challenges of chronic pain and the setbacks that can occur along the way. Developing resilience involves a combination of psychological strategies, healthy lifestyle choices, and support systems that work together to empower individuals to manage their pain effectively.

Anticipate Pain Flare-Ups

Managing chronic pain can be unpredictable, and despite your best efforts, there will inevitably be times when your pain intensifies—these are known as pain flare-ups. It's important to recognize that flare-ups are a normal part of living with chronic pain, and they do not necessarily mean that you've done something wrong or that new damage has occurred in your body.

Understanding and accepting that flare-ups will happen can help reduce the stress and anxiety that often accompany them. Instead of being caught off guard, you can approach these moments with a sense of preparedness. This mindset shift allows you to focus on managing the flare-up rather than worrying about its occurrence. By anticipating flare-ups, you position yourself to proactively engage with your pain management strategies, ensuring you are better equipped to handle these challenging periods.

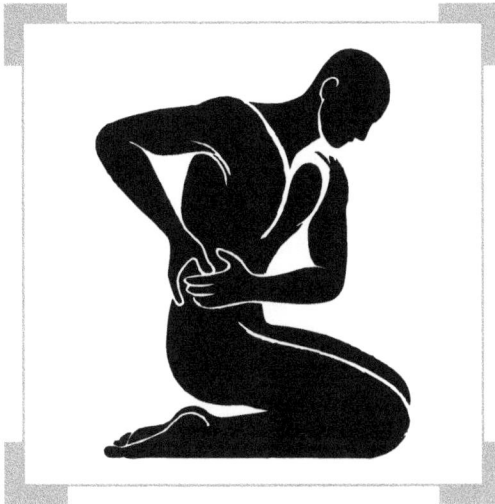

Managing Pain Flare-Ups

When a flare-up occurs, it's natural to feel overwhelmed, and using your pain management tools might seem more difficult. However, during these high-pain moments, your coping skills are most crucial. These skills are your first line of defense against worsening your symptoms, helping to mitigate the impact of the flare-up on your daily life.

To effectively manage flare-ups, practicing these coping strategies is essential even when you're not in pain. This consistent practice helps to ingrain these techniques into your daily routine, making them second nature. When these skills become habits, you'll find it easier to access them during a flare-up, even when your pain is at its peak.

Key flare-up management strategies might include deep breathing exercises, progressive muscle relaxation, pacing yourself, distraction techniques, or mindfulness meditation. Over time, regular practice of these methods will enhance your ability to respond to pain flare-ups with resilience and calm.

Additionally, it's important to remember that self-compassion plays a significant role in coping with flare-ups. Acknowledge your efforts and recognize that managing pain is a process. By staying committed to using your coping tools and practicing them regularly, you build a strong foundation for handling flare-ups effectively. This proactive approach helps you manage pain more successfully and empowers you to maintain a higher quality of life, even in the face of chronic pain.

Plan to manage a flare-up.

When in a flare-up, it is often difficult to think about the tools and strategies in your 'toolbox' to support you in managing it. The table below is not exclusive, and again, writing this down before a flare-up allows you to refer back to this when it is needed and reminds you of some of the strategies that have worked for you in the past.

Strategies to minimize flare-up intensity, for example, take a stretch break.

Consider the following: Medicines - Physical activity – Rest - Meditation/ relaxation.

- Healthcare team support - Family, friends and work

If I experience a pain flare-up, I will focus on the following actions for the next few hours: (e.g., engage in relaxation techniques and practice deep breathing)

If I experience a pain flare-up, I will adjust my activities over the next few days as follows: (e.g., reduce my activity level without stopping completely)

Plan to Get Back on Track: (e.g., resume activity by starting a walking program for 10 minutes a day, making sure to use my pacing techniques)

I will treat myself once the flare-up subsides (e.g., enjoying some extra time with my friends)

Building Mental and Emotional Strength

- <u>Mindfulness Practices:</u> Mindfulness involves staying present at the moment and acknowledging thoughts and feelings without judgment. Techniques such as mindful breathing, body scans, and mindful observation help reduce stress and anxiety, which are often exacerbated by chronic pain. Individuals can break the cycle of negative thoughts that can worsen pain perception by focusing on the here and now.

- Meditation, whether guided by an instructor or self-led, is crucial in promoting relaxation and mental clarity. Regular meditation practices can help quiet the mind, reduce stress hormones, and create a mental space where pain does not dominate one's consciousness. Over time, meditation helps build a more resilient mindset, making it easier to cope with the ups and downs of chronic pain.

- Cognitive Behavioral Therapy (CBT): Thought Pattern Changes: CBT is a psychological approach that focuses on altering negative thought patterns that can contribute to feelings of helplessness or hopelessness in the face of chronic pain. By learning to identify and challenge these thoughts, individuals can shift their mindset towards more positive, constructive thinking that supports resilience.

- Behavioral Adjustments: CBT also involves modifying behaviors that may exacerbate pain. This could include learning to pace oneself during activities, avoiding overexertion, and finding new ways to engage in enjoyable activities that don't trigger pain. These adjustments help create a more balanced and sustainable approach to daily life.

- Support Networks:

- Social Support: Building a strong family, friends, and peers network is essential for emotional resilience. These relationships provide encouragement, understanding, and practical support, helping individuals feel less isolated in their pain management journey. Engaging with support groups, whether in person or online, can also offer a sense of community and shared experience that is invaluable for resilience.

- Professional Support: Accessing mental health professionals, such as therapists or counselors, provides additional support. These professionals can offer guidance, coping strategies, and emotional support tailored to the unique challenges of chronic pain, helping individuals build and maintain their resilience over time.

Healthy Coping Strategies

- *Stress Management:*

- Deep Breathing: Deep breathing exercises are a simple yet effective way to calm the mind and body. By focusing on slow, controlled breaths, individuals can lower their heart rate, reduce muscle tension, and shift their focus away from pain. These exercises can be practiced anywhere and are a powerful tool for managing stress.

- <u>Yoga and Stretching:</u> Incorporating yoga and stretching into a daily routine helps reduce stress, flexibility, and muscle tension. Yoga, in particular, combines physical postures with breathing exercises and meditation, offering a holistic approach to managing both physical and emotional aspects of pain.

-   <u>Progressive Muscle Relaxation</u>: This technique involves systematically tensing and relaxing different muscle groups in the body. By doing so, individuals can become more aware of where they hold tension and learn to release it, reducing pain and promoting a sense of relaxation.

- *Positive Lifestyle Choices:*

- <u>Physical Activity</u>: Regular physical activity, tailored to individual capabilities, is crucial for managing chronic pain and building resilience. Exercise releases endorphins, the body's natural painkillers, and helps maintain overall physical health, essential for coping with pain.

- <u>Balanced Diet:</u> Nutrition plays a key role in pain management. A balanced diet rich in anti-inflammatory foods, such as fruits, vegetables, whole grains, and lean proteins, supports overall health and can help reduce pain and inflammation. Proper nutrition also contributes to mental well-being, which is vital for resilience.

- <u>Adequate Sleep:</u> Ensuring restful sleep is fundamental to managing pain and maintaining a positive outlook. Poor sleep can exacerbate pain and make it harder to cope with daily challenges. Establishing a regular sleep routine, creating a comfortable sleep environment, and addressing any sleep issues, such as insomnia or sleep apnea, are important steps in building resilience.

Resilience Training

- <u>Mental Toughness Programs</u>: These programs focus on exercises and activities designed to build psychological resilience. They might include challenges that push individuals to develop problem-solving skills, adaptability, and persistence. Over time, these activities help strengthen mental toughness, making it easier to face and overcome the challenges associated with chronic pain.

- Emotional resilience involves strategies to maintain a positive outlook even in the face of setbacks. This might include practicing gratitude, staying connected with loved ones, and engaging in activities that bring joy and fulfillment. Emotional resilience is about recognizing that while setbacks are inevitable, they are not insurmountable.

Long-Term Maintenance

- Regular Check-Ups:

  - Follow-Ups: Routine visits to healthcare providers are essential for monitoring progress and making necessary adjustments to the pain management plan. Regular check-ups allow for early detection of new issues and ensure the treatment plan remains effective.

  - Adjustments: As progress is made, adjustments to the pain management plan may be necessary. This could involve modifying exercises, changing medications, or introducing new therapies. Flexibility in the treatment approach is key to maintaining long-term health and resilience.

- Ongoing Education:

  - Staying Informed: Maintaining the latest pain management techniques and therapies is crucial for ongoing success. This might involve reading books, attending workshops, or consulting healthcare providers about new options. Being well-informed empowers individuals to make proactive decisions about their health.

- Adaptation and Adjustment:

  - Flexible Strategies: Life is dynamic, and so is pain management. Continuously adapting and adjusting strategies to fit changing conditions and challenges is essential. This might mean altering exercise routines, trying new pain relief methods, or adjusting lifestyle habits. The ability to adapt is a core component of resilience.

Tracking and Progress Monitoring

- Pain Diary: A pain diary provides a structured format for tracking pain levels, triggers, and relief measures. Keeping a diary helps individuals identify patterns in their pain, making it easier to manage and anticipate pain episodes.

  - Regular Entries: Consistently documenting pain experiences daily or weekly provides valuable insights into what works and what doesn't. This information can be shared with healthcare providers to fine-tune treatment plans.

- Progress Evaluation:

- <u>Assessments:</u> Regular evaluations are crucial for measuring pain, function, and overall health improvements. These assessments provide a clear picture of how far an individual has come and what needs to be addressed.

- <u>Adjustments:</u> Based on assessment results, informed changes can be made to the action plan. This might involve setting new goals, introducing different therapies, or adjusting current treatments to meet the individual's needs better.

- Goal Setting and Achievement:

- <u>Realistic Goals</u>: Helping patients set achievable and meaningful goals is an important process. Realistic goals keep individuals motivated and focused on their progress.

- <u>Celebrating Milestones:</u> Recognizing and celebrating progress and achievements, no matter how small, is vital for maintaining motivation and a positive outlook. Each milestone reached is a step closer to improved well-being.

Resources and Support

<u>- Further Reading:</u>

- Books: Suggested titles on pain management and physiotherapy provide additional insights and strategies for managing chronic pain.

- Websites: Reputable online resources offer access to up-to-date information and support for those dealing with chronic pain.

- Articles: Research articles and informative pieces on pain management help individuals stay informed about the latest developments in the field.

<u>- Support Networks:</u>

- Support Groups: Information on local and online support groups for chronic pain sufferers provides opportunities for connection and shared experience.

- Community Resources: Access to community programs and services for pain management can provide additional support and resources for individuals on their pain management journey.

- Staying Motivated:

Encouragement: Tips and strategies for staying motivated and committed to the pain management journey are essential for long-term success. Encouragement might come from setting new goals, finding new interests, or connecting with others who understand the journey.

Maintaining a positive mindset throughout the process is crucial. It's important to remember that setbacks are a part of the journey and that persistence and resilience can lead to significant improvements over time. Summarizing key points and the holistic approach to pain management reinforces the importance of addressing both physical and emotional aspects of pain.

As you reach the end of this workbook, it's important to remember that the journey toward pain management and improved quality of life doesn't end here. The ongoing self-management and resilience principles discussed throughout these chapters are key to sustaining long-term well-being. By integrating the strategies of pain relief, recovery, rehabilitation, and resilience into your daily life, you are empowered to take control of your health. With the knowledge and tools provided in this book, you are well-equipped to continue your journey toward lasting wellness and a life defined by strength and self-empowerment.

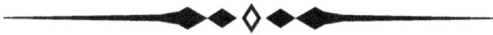

BIBLIOGRAPHY

Abdoli, J., Motamedi, S. A., & Zargaran, A. (2019). A Short Review on the History of Anesthesia in Ancient Civilizations. *Journal of Research on History of Medicine, 8*(3), 147-156. Retrieved 8 15, 2023, from https://doaj.org/article/38e9ad035c854f2eabedaba33feafe9d

Amris K, B. C. (2019). The benefit of adding a physiotherapy or occupational therapy intervention programme to a standardized group-based interdisciplinary rehabilitation programme for patients with chronic widespread pain: a randomized active-controlled non-blinded trial. *Clinical Rehabilitation, 33*(8), 1367-1381. doi:10.1177/0269215519843986

Andrews NE, S. J. (2015). Overactivity in chronic pain: Is it a valid construct? *Pain Journal*, 1991-2000. doi:10.1097/j.pain.0000000000000259

Bannister, K. (2019). Descending pain modulation: influence and impact. *Current Opinion in Physiology, 11*, 62-66. Retrieved 8 18, 2023, from https://sciencedirect.com/science/article/pii/s2468867319301117

Brosseau L, T. J.-A. (2017, May). The Ottawa panel clinical practice guidelines for the management of knee osteoarthritis. Part three: aerobic exercise programs. *Clin Rehabil*, 612-624. doi:10.1177/0269215517691085. Epub 2017 Feb 9. PMID: 28183194.

Cagnie, B., Coppieters, I., Denecker, S., Six, J., Danneels, L., Meeus, M., & Meeus, M. (2014). Central sensitization in fibromyalgia? A systematic review on structural and functional brain MRI. *Seminars in Arthritis and Rheumatism, 44*(1), 68-75. Retrieved 8 18, 2023, from https://sciencedirect.com/science/article/pii/s004901721400002x

Calder, P. C. (2013). Omega-3 polyunsaturated fatty acids and inflammatory processes: Nutrition or pharmacology? *British Journal of Clinical Pharmacology, 75*(3), 645-662.

Cascella, M. M. (2022). Pathophysiology of Nociception and Rare Genetic Disorders with Increased Pain Threshold or Pain Insensitivity. *Pathophysiology, 29*(3). doi:https://doi.org/10.3390/pathophysiology29030035

Cosio D, D. A. (2020). Adherence and Relapse – How to Maintain Long-Term Gains in Patients with Chronic Conditions. *Pract Pain Manag, 20*(6), issue 6.

Davidson, R. J., Kabat-Zinn, J., Schumacher, J. R., Rosenkranz, M. A., Muller, D., Santorelli, S. F., . . . Sheridan, J. F. (2003). Alterations in Brain and Immune Function Produced by Mindfulness Meditation. *Psychosomatic Medicine, 65*(4), 564-570. Retrieved 6 9, 2024, from https://ncbi.nlm.nih.gov/pubmed/12883106

Denneny, D., Frijdal, A., Bianchi-Berthouze, N., Greenwood, J., McLoughlin, R., Petersen, K., & Singh, A. (2020, March). The application of psychologically informed practice: observations of experienced physiotherapists working with people with chronic pain. *Physiotherapy, 106*, 163-173. doi:10.1016/j.physio.2019.01.014

DeSantana, J. M., Walsh, D. M., Vance, C., Rakel, B. A., & Sluka, K. A. (2008). Effectiveness of transcutaneous electrical nerve stimulation for treatment of hyperalgesia and pain. *Current Rheumatology Reports, 10*(6), 492-499. Retrieved 8 16, 2023, from https://ncbi.nlm.nih.gov/pmc/articles/pmc2746624

Dolbier, C. L., & Rush, T. E. (2012). Efficacy of Abbreviated Progressive Muscle Relaxation in a High-Stress College Sample. *International Journal of Stress Management, 19*(1), 48-68. Retrieved 6 12, 2024, from https://psycnet.apa.org/record/2012-04979-002

Dwyer, C. P., Durand, H., MacNeela, P., Reynolds, B., Hamm, R. M., Main, C. J., . . . McGuire, B. E. (2016). Effectiveness of a biopsychosocial e-learning intervention on the clinical judgements of medical students and GP trainees regarding future risk of disability in patients with chronic lower back pain: study protocol for a randomised controlled trial. *BMJ Open, 6*(5). Retrieved 8 18, 2023, from https://ncbi.nlm.nih.gov/pubmed/27231000

Eccleston, C. (2001). Role of psychology in pain management. *BJA: British Journal of Anaesthesia, 87*(1), 144-152. Retrieved 10 8, 2023, from https://academic.oup.com/bja/article/87/1/144/304231

Ello-Martin JA, L. J. (2005, July). The influence of food portion size and energy density on energy intake: implications for weight management. *Am J Clin Nutr*, 236S-241S. doi: doi: 10.1093/ajcn/82.1.236S. PMID: 16002828.

Elma Ö, B. K. (2022, October). The Importance of Nutrition as a Lifestyle Factor in Chronic Pain Management: A Narrative Review. *J Clin Med, 11*(19), 5950. doi:10.1093/ajcn/82.1.236S. PMID: 16002828.

Halliday MH, G. A. (2019, April). Treatment Effect Sizes of Mechanical Diagnosis and Therapy for Pain and Disability in Patients With Low Back Pain: A Systematic Review. *J Orthop Sports Phys Ther*, 219-229. doi:10.2519/jospt.2019.8734. Epub 2019 Feb 13. PMID: 30759358.

Hammond, D. C. (2008). Hypnosis as Sole Anesthesia for Major Surgeries: Historical & Contemporary Perspectives. *American Journal of Clinical Hypnosis, 51*(2), 101-121. Retrieved 8 16, 2023, from https://ncbi.nlm.nih.gov/pubmed/18998378

Hartrick CT, D. A. (2023, January). Pain 360: Emerging topics in the pathophysiology, diagnosis, and treatment of chronic pain. (S. Marchand, Ed.) *Front. Pain Res.* doi:https://doi.org/10.3389/fpain.2022.1123272

Hefford, C. (2008). McKenzie classification of mechanical spinal pain: Profile of syndromes and directions of preference. *Manual Therapy, 13*(1), 75-81. doi:https://doi.org/10.1016/j.math.2006.08.005

Hempel, S. e. (2012). Probiotics for the prevention and treatment of antibiotic-associated diarrhea: A systematic review and meta-analysis. *JAMA, 307*(18), 1959-1969.

Heyl, J. d. (2005). Handbook of pain management, Ronald Melzack, Patrick D. Wall : book review. *Southern African Journal of Anaesthesia and Analgesia, 11*(1), 38. Retrieved 8 15, 2023, from https://journals.co.za/content/medsajaa/11/1/ejc73456

Ho, H. (2007). From Descartes to fMRI. Pain theories and pain concepts. *Schmerz, 21*(4), 307. Retrieved 8 15, 2023, from https://ncbi.nlm.nih.gov/pubmed/17674057

Hu, F. B. (2013). Resolved: There is sufficient scientific evidence that decreasing sugar-sweetened beverage consumption will reduce the prevalence of obesity and obesity-related diseases. *Obesity Reviews, 14*(8), 606.

IASP. (n.d.). Retrieved from https://www.iasp-pain.org/resources/terminology/#pain

Jacob B. Lindheimer, A. J.-S. (2019). Influence of pain anticipation on brain activity and pain perception in Gulf War Veterans with chronic musculoskeletal pain. *International Journal of Psychophysiology, 56*(12). doi: https://doi.org/10.1111/psyp.13452

Jenkins, D. J. (2002). Glycemic index: Overview of implications in health and disease. *American Journal of Clinical Nutrition, 76(1), , 76*(1), 266S-273S.

Katz, J., & Rosenbloom, B. N. (2015). The golden anniversary of Melzack and Wall's gate control theory of pain: Celebrating 50 years of pain research and management. *Pain Research & Management, 20*(6), 285-286. Retrieved 8 15, 2023, from https://ncbi.nlm.nih.gov/pubmed/26642069

Kempermann, G., Fabel, K., Ehninger, D., Babu, H., Leal-Galicia, P., Garthe, A., & Wolf, S. A. (2010). Why and How Physical Activity Promotes Experience-Induced Brain Plasticity. *Frontiers in Neuroscience, 4*, 189-189. Retrieved 6 9, 2024, from https://frontiersin.org/articles/10.3389/fnins.2010.00189/full

Lema, I. C. (2020). What's new in chronic pain pathophysiology. *Canadian Journal of Pain, 4*(4), 13-18. doi:10.1080/24740527.2020.1752641

Lewis, J., Green, A., & Wright, C. (2005). Subacromial impingement syndrome: the role of posture and muscle imbalance. *Journal of Shoulder and Elbow Surgery, 14*(4), 385-392. Retrieved 6 10, 2024, from https://ncbi.nlm.nih.gov/pubmed/16015238

Lim JA, C. S. (2018, June). Cognitive-behavioral therapy for patients with chronic pain: Implications of gender differences in empathy. *Medicine*, 97. doi:10.1097/MD.0000000000010867

Liu X, L. L. (2014). Memory impairment in chronic pain patients and the related neuropsychological mechanisms: a review. *Acta Neuropsychiatr, 26*(4), 195-201. doi:10.1017/neu.2013.47. PMID: 25279415.

Louw, A., Diener, I., Butler, D. S., & Puentedura, E. J. (2011). The Effect of Neuroscience Education on Pain, Disability, Anxiety, and Stress in Chronic Musculoskeletal Pain. *Archives of Physical Medicine and Rehabilitation, 92*(12), 2041-2056. Retrieved 6 9, 2024, from https://archives-pmr.org/article/s0003-9993(11)00670-8/fulltext

Macintyre, P. (2001). Safety and efficacy of patient-controlled analgesia. *BJA: British Journal of Anaesthesia, 87*(1), 36-46. Retrieved 8 15, 2023, from https://academic.oup.com/bja/article/87/1/36/304220

Makki, K. e. (2018). The impact of dietary fiber on gut microbiota in host health and disease. *Cell Host & Microbe, 23*(6), 705-715.

Marchand, S. (2014). *Neurophysiology of Pain*. Retrieved 8 15, 2023, from https://link.springer.com/chapter/10.1007/978-2-8178-0414-9_3

May, S., Nanche, G., & Pingle, S. (2011). High frequency of McKenzie's postural syndrome in young population of non-care seeking individuals. *Journal of Manual & Manipulative Therapy, 19*(1), 48-54. Retrieved 6 10, 2024, from https://ncbi.nlm.nih.gov/pmc/articles/pmc3172957

McCallie, M. S., Blum, C. M., & Hood, C. J. (2006). Progressive Muscle Relaxation. *Journal of Human Behavior in The Social Environment, 13*(3), 51-66. Retrieved 6 12, 2024, from https://tandfonline.com/doi/abs/10.1300/j137v13n03_04

Megan Pomarensky, M. C., Luciana Macedo, P. P., & Lisa C. Carlesso, P. P. (2022). Management of Chronic Musculoskeletal Pain Through a Biopsychosocial Lens. *J Athl Train*, 57 (4): 312–318. doi:https://doi.org/10.4085/1062-6050-0521.20

Meise R, C. G. (2023). Additional effects of pain neuroscience education combined with physiotherapy on the headache frequency of adult patients with migraine: A randomized controlled trial. *Cephalalgia*. doi:10.1177/03331024221144781

Meldrum, M. L. (2003). A Capsule History of Pain Management. *JAMA, 290*(18), 2470-2475. Retrieved 8 15, 2023, from https://jamanetwork.com/journals/jama/fullarticle/197633

Melzack, R. (2005). Evolution of the neuromatrix theory of pain. The Prithvi Raj Lecture: presented at the third World Congress of World Institute of Pain, Barcelona 2004. *Pain Practice, 5*(2), 85-94. Retrieved 8 18, 2023, from https://ncbi.nlm.nih.gov/pubmed/17177754

Mendell, L. M. (2014). Constructing and deconstructing the gate theory of pain. *Pain, 155*(2), 210-216. Retrieved 8 16, 2023, from https://ncbi.nlm.nih.gov/pmc/articles/pmc4009371

Moayedi, M., Davis, K. D., & Davis, K. D. (2013). Theories of pain: from specificity to gate control. *Journal of Neurophysiology, 109*(1), 5-12. Retrieved 8 16, 2023, from https://physiology.org/doi/full/10.1152/jn.00457.2012

Moriarty, O., McGuire, B. E., & Finn, D. P. (2011). The effect of pain on cognitive function: a review of clinical and preclinical research. *Progress in Neurobiology, 93*(3), 385-404. Retrieved 8 22, 2023, from https://sciencedirect.com/science/article/pii/s0301008211000037

Moseley, G. (2004). Graded motor imagery is effective for long-standing complex regional pain syndrome: a randomised controlled trial. *Pain, 108*(1), 192-198. Retrieved 6 9, 2024, from https://ncbi.nlm.nih.gov/pubmed/15109523

Nuttall, F. Q. (1991). Plasma glucose and insulin responses to macronutrients in nondiabetic and NIDDM subjects. *Diabetes Care, 14*(9), 824-838.

Offenbaecher, M. (2021, March 05). Pain is not the major determinant of quality of life in fibromyalgia: results from a retrospective "real world" data analysis of fibromyalgia patients. *Rheumatology International*, 41, pages1995–2006 (2021). doi:https://doi.org/10.1007/s00296-020-04702-5

Pandey, K. B. (2009). Plant polyphenols as dietary antioxidants in human health and disease. *Oxidative Medicine and Cellular Longevity, 2*(5), 270-278.

Pérez-Belmonte, L. M. (2018). Role of antioxidants in the pathophysiology of chronic pain conditions. *Antioxidants, 7*(10), 121.

Petersen-Felix, S., & Curatolo, M. (2002). Neuroplasticity - An important factor in acute and chronic pain. *Swiss Medical Weekly, 132*(2122), 273-278. Retrieved 6 9, 2024, from https://ncbi.nlm.nih.gov/pubmed/12362284

R, S. (1985). Friedrich Wilhelm Sertürner and the discovery of morphine. *Pharmacy in history, 27*(2), 61. Retrieved 8 15, 2023, from https://ncbi.nlm.nih.gov/pubmed/11611724

R.Mulligan, B. (2010). *Manual therapy NAGS,SNAGS,MWMS 6th edition.*

Roditi, D., & Robinson, M. E. (2011). The role of psychological interventions in the management of patients with chronic pain. *Psychology Research and Behavior Management, 4*, 41-49. Retrieved 10 8, 2023, from https://ncbi.nlm.nih.gov/pmc/articles/pmc3218789

Rosenblum, A., Marsch, L. A., Joseph, H., & Portenoy, R. K. (2008). Opioids and the Treatment of Chronic Pain: Controversies, Current Status, and Future Directions. *Experimental and Clinical Psychopharmacology, 16*(5), 405-416. Retrieved 8 15, 2023, from https://ncbi.nlm.nih.gov/pmc/articles/pmc2711509

Rouch, I., Edjolo, A., Laurent, B., Pongan, E., Dartigues, J.-F., & Amieva, H. (2023, February). Association between chronic pain and long-term cognitive decline in a population-based cohort of elderly participants. *PAIN, 162*(2), 552-560. doi:10.1097/j.pain.0000000000002047

Sator-Katzenschlager, S. M. (2014). Pain and neuroplasticity. *Revista Médica Clínica Las Condes, 25*(4), 699-706. Retrieved 6 9, 2024, from https://sciencedirect.com/science/article/pii/s0716864014700914

Seamark, D. (2015). Books: The Story of Pain: From Prayer to Painkillers: Agony's Journey. *British Journal of General Practice, 65*(632), 146-146. Retrieved 8 15, 2023, from https://bjgp.org/content/65/632/146.1

Siddall, P. J., & Siddall, P. J. (2013). Neuroplasticity and pain: what does it all mean? *The Medical Journal of Australia, 198*(4), 177-178. Retrieved 6 9,

2024, from https://mja.com.au/journal/2013/198/4/neuroplasticity-and-pain-what-does-it-all-mean

Slavin, J. (2013). Fiber and prebiotics: Mechanisms and health benefits. *Nutrients, 5*(4), 1417-1435.

Solé, E., Racine, M., Tomé-Pires, C., Galán, S., Jensen, M. P., & Miró, J. (2022, May). Social Factors, Disability, and Depressive Symptoms in Adults With Chronic Pain. *The Clinical Journal of Pain, 36*(5), 371-378. doi:10.1097/AJP.0000000000000815

Takasaki H, O. K. (2017). Inter-examiner classification reliability of Mechanical Diagnosis and Therapy for extremity problems - Systematic review. *Musculoskelet Sci Pract*, 78-84. doi:10.1016/j.msksp.2016.12.016. Epub 2017 Jan 5. PMID: 28637606.

Todd, J., Clarke, P., Hughes, A. M., & van Ryckeghem, D. (2023, March). Attentional bias malleability as a predictor of daily pain interference. *PAIN, 164*(3), 598-604. doi:10.1097/j.pain.0000000000002744

Wilson JM, H. I. (2023, January 7). The role of dispositional mindfulness in the fear-avoidance model of pain. *PLoS ONE 18(1): e0280740.* doi:https://doi.org/10.1371/journal.pone.0280740

Wong, W. S., Lam, H. M., Chen, P. P., Chow, Y. F., Wong, S., Lim, H. S., . . . Fielding, R. (2015). The Fear-Avoidance Model of Chronic Pain: Assessing the Role of Neuroticism and Negative Affect in Pain Catastrophizing Using Structural Equation Modeling. *International Journal of Behavioral Medicine, 22*(1), 118-131. Retrieved 8 18, 2023, from https://link.springer.com/article/10.1007/s12529-014-9413-7

Woznowski-Vu, A. M., Uddin, Z. P., Flegg, D. B., Aternali, A. B., Wickens, R. M., Sullivan, M. J., . . . Wideman, T. H. (2019, August). Comparing Novel and Existing Measures of Sensitivity to Physical Activity Among People With Chronic Musculoskeletal Pain: The Importance of Tailoring Activity to Pain. *The Clinical Journal of Pain*, 656-667. doi:10.1097/AJP.0000000000000732

www.ingramcontent.com/pod-product-compliance
Lightning Source LLC
Chambersburg PA
CBHW052017030426
42335CB00026B/3183